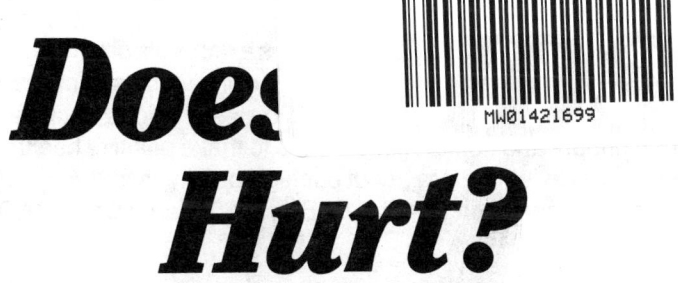

Does It Hurt?
Educating Young Children About AIDS

SECOND EDITION

Marcia Quackenbush, MS, MFCC
Sylvia Villarreal, MD

Suggestions for parents, teachers and other care providers of children to age 10

ETR ASSOCIATES
Santa Cruz, California
1992

ETR Associates (Education, Training and Research) is a nonprofit organization committed to fostering the health, well-being and cultural diversity of individuals, families, schools and communities. The publishing program of ETR Associates provides books and materials that empower young people and adults with the skills to make positive health choices. We invite health professionals to learn more about our high-quality resources and our training and research programs by contacting us at P.O. Box 1830, Santa Cruz, CA 95061-1830.

© 1988 by ETR Associates. Second edition © 1992.
All rights reserved. Published by ETR Associates,
P.O. Box 1830, Santa Cruz, CA 95061-1830.

10 9 8 7 6 5

Printed in the United States of America

Illustrations by Marcia Quackenbush
Design by Ann Smiley and Julia Chiapella

Library of Congress Cataloging-in-Publication Data

Quackenbush, Marcia.
    Does AIDS hurt? : educating young children about AIDS : suggestions for parents, teachers, and other care providers of children to age 10 / Marcia Quackenbush, Sylvia Villarreal. — 2nd ed.
        p. cm.
    Includes bibliographical references.
    ISBN 1-56071-084-5
    1. AIDS (Disease)—Popular works. 2. Child rearing.
3. Health education (Elementary). I. Villarreal, Sylvia. II. Title.
RC607.A26Q29   1992
616.97'92—dc20   92-25691

Contents

Acknowledgments   vii

Preface   ix

Notes to the Reader   xiii

SECTION 1   HIV AND YOUNG CHILDREN

Chapter 1.   Talking with Young Children About AIDS   3
    Why Do Young Children Need to Know About AIDS and HIV?   6
    Comprehensive School Health Programs   7
    Additional HIV Prevention Strategies for Young Children   9
    Keeping Parents Involved   9
    Talking About HIV: What Do You Need to Know?   10
    Four Important Values When Providing HIV Information   11

Chapter 2.   Things to Keep in Mind   13
    Four Goals for Parents, Teachers and Caretakers   15
    Teaching Children About Sexuality   16
    Give Yourself Some Leeway! Basic Guidelines   16
    The Meaning Behind the Question   17

Chapter 3.   What Are Children Asking and How Can You Answer Them?   23
    General Things to Keep in Mind   25
    Suggested Steps in Answering Children's Questions   26
    Questions and Answers   26

Chapter 4. When Should You Bring Up the Topic? 41
    Circumstances in Which You May Want to Bring Up AIDS 42

Chapter 5. Special Circumstances: When a Child, Family or Friends Are at Risk for or Infected with HIV 47
    Tinisha: Having a Mother with HIV-Related Illnesses 51
    Lucas: A Boy with AIDS 54
    Jackie: Having a Father at Risk 58

Chapter 6. Issues for the Young Child in Foster Care 63

Chapter 7. AIDS Education in the Early Elementary Classroom 67
    Specific Content About AIDS That Young Children Should Understand 68
    Classroom Examples: Integrating HIV Education with Other Lessons 70
        A Kindergarten Class 70
        A Second-Grade Class 72
        A Fourth-Grade Class 76
    Developing AIDS-Specific Curricula for Younger Children 81

Chapter 8. Trouble-Shooting: Anticipating Problems That Might Come Up in Discussing AIDS with Young Children 85

Chapter 9. How to Do It Right: The School with HIV-Infected Students or Staff 91
    Groundwork 92
    If and When It Happens: Informing Teachers, Parents, Students and the Community at Large 93
    Our Imaginary Community 94
        What Happened 94
        What Was Taught to the Early Elementary Students 96
        Class Discussion Outline 97

SECTION 2   BACKGROUND INFORMATION

Chapter 10.   HIV Information: Answers for Adults   101
    General Information   102
    More Questions About Transmission   105
    More Information About HIV and AIDS   111
    Doubts About Casual Transmission   119
    Further Information   122

Chapter 11.   Staying Updated on HIV Information   123

Chapter 12.   HIV Information and Developmental Stages:
    What Do Children Want to Know About AIDS, When?   125
        Infants (birth to 11 months)   126
        Toddlers   127
        Early Childhood   128
        School Age   131

Chapter 13.   Signs of Child Sexual Abuse   137
    Indicators of Sexual Abuse in Children   137
        Physical Signs   138
        Behavior/Attitudinal Signs   138

SECTION 3   FURTHER RESOURCES

Appendix A: Readings   143

Appendix B: Information Sources   147

Acknowledgments

Many people have contributed time, expertise, suggestions and support in the writing of this book. We could never have included the breadth of experience and knowledge we have here without their help. We want to thank the individuals who helped us develop our concepts and who read drafts at various stages, improving it with many useful comments. These include:

Donna Berka
Paul Fishman, MD
Frances Kendall, PhD
JoAnn Loulan, MA, MFCC
Mary McDonald
Renetia Martin, MSW, LCSW
Cheri Pies, MSW, MPH
JoAnna Rinaldi
David Schonfeld, MD
Debra Singer, MD
Ellen Wagman, MPH
Debra Zilavy, RN, MS, MFCC

We also appreciate the general support of Moses Grossman, M.D.

Very special thanks are due our editors, Mary Nelson and Kay Clark. They have certainly influenced this work, advising us with seemingly limitless patience and wisdom, encouraging us with enthusiasm, and bringing order out of chaos with their excellent sense of syntax.

Kathleen Middleton, MS, CHES, spent time above and beyond the call of duty helping us develop our chapter on *AIDS Education in the Early Elementary Classroom,* and for this we are deeply grateful.

Finally, we want to thank the many parents, teachers, health providers, and other professionals, who have shared their questions and experiences willingly and helpfully; and the children themselves, who so often touch our hearts and make our work the reward that it is.

Preface

It has been five years since we started working on the first edition of *Does AIDS Hurt?* In that time, many things about the HIV epidemic have changed, while other matters remain much as they were in 1987. In the area of HIV education for young children, we have also seen some things change and others remain fairly constant.

The HIV Epidemic

When this book first went to press, 60,000 cases of AIDS had been reported in the United States. Today as we write this new preface, that number is over 200,000. By the time you read this, the number will be higher still. The magnitude of the epidemic is continuing to increase.

Treatments for HIV were mostly experimental five years ago, and of questionable value. Today, there are medications which are known to slow the progression of the disease. There are preventive treatments for several illnesses common in people with HIV. There is hope now that treatments will continue to improve, and that people with HIV will one day have a condition that is "manageable," in the same way diabetes and high blood pressure are today.

The human face of the epidemic has also changed over the past five years. Today, there are greater numbers of injection drug users being diagnosed. The sexual partners and children of injection drug users are also being diagnosed with AIDS. In fact, nearly one in three cases of AIDS can be traced directly or indirectly to injection drug use.

There are also more women, more heterosexuals, more people of color and more youth being diagnosed with AIDS.

The federal government may be revising the definition of AIDS shortly after this book goes to press. This more inclusive definition gives many people an AIDS diagnosis who were considered before to have "symptomatic HIV infection." This change may add an additional 100,000 cases of AIDS to the toll, further burdening already overwhelmed health providers and increasing the demands on local and state health departments.

More people in the public eye have acknowledged having HIV or AIDS. We have heard of actors, writers, newscasters, musicians, politicians and athletes with HIV. Reports on these individuals appear in magazines and newspapers. Their personal stories come into our homes on television broadcasts. Most of us have a greater familiarity with HIV today than we did five years ago.

The HIV epidemic will be with us for a long time—very possibly for the rest of our lives. It is a fact of life we must all learn to live with, and one we must teach our children to live with as well.

Educating Young Children About HIV and AIDS

In 1987, when we were writing the first edition of this book, the suggestion that adults should talk with young children about AIDS seemed extreme to many. "Why would anyone want to talk about AIDS with young children? Don't children already have enough to worry about?" people asked us.

Today, more teachers, parents and others who work with children have had experiences which underscore the main premise of our first edition: *Children do have questions about AIDS. If you are willing to answer these questions, you can help children in important ways.* The thought of a young child asking about AIDS seems less strange, and the need to answer that question clearer, than was the case a few years back.

We agree that children today have a lot on their minds, and they certainly don't need new things to fear. This is exactly the reason it is so important to respond to their questions about AIDS. Children have heard about AIDS. They may be afraid of "catching" it themselves, or they may worry about their parents contracting the disease. They may have come across stories of children with AIDS who have been abandoned or mistreated. They may have picked up perplexing (and perhaps inaccurate) information about AIDS, sexuality and drug use from schoolmates. They need reassurance, accurate information and acceptance from the caring adults around them to better master this confusing situation.

We wrote this book because we wanted to support parents, teachers and others in guiding children through life with one less fear. Helping children understand AIDS in a productive and useful manner, appropriate to their age, is one of the many challenges faced in this endeavor. We hope this book will prove useful to people who are facing this challenge in the years ahead.

We dedicate this book to children, who are our future.

Notes to the Reader

1. A number of vignettes are included in this book. We have changed the names and some of the identifying information in these stories to protect the confidentiality of the persons involved.
2. When we refer to "young children" in this book, we are speaking of children up to age ten.
3. There are two terms readers will want to be familiar with for this book to be most helpful.

    AIDS: A disease which involves damage to the immune system, making a person susceptible to a number of serious diseases which do not affect people with healthy immune systems.

    HIV: *Human immunodeficiency virus,* the virus which causes AIDS. A person may be infected with HIV for many years without having signs or symptoms of illness.

    People with HIV infection may fall anywhere along a spectrum of illness. Some have no symptoms. Some have physical symptoms, but do not meet the criteria for an AIDS diagnosis. Others have physical symptoms and do meet the criteria for an AIDS diagnosis. And some may have no physical symptoms, but have laboratory values (based on certain blood tests) which meet the criteria for an AIDS diagnosis.

Young children (especially those under nine years) generally will not make these finer distinctions between HIV and AIDS. They may ask questions about "AIDS," for example, when the term "HIV infection" would be more accurate. We need to keep our explanations as simple as possible for young children, however. We feel it is acceptable to sacrifice some points of scientific accuracy so we may better clarify more general and essential concepts to young children.

In this book, we have used the term "AIDS" when discussing children's questions ("When young children ask about AIDS, we will want to give simple, truthful answers"). We use "AIDS" in most of our sample answers for children (see Chapter 3: *What Are Children Asking and How Can You Answer Them?*). We also use "AIDS" when describing the sp,ecific medical condition of an AIDS diagnosis. In most other contexts, we use the term "HIV" or "HIV infection."

SECTION 1

HIV AND YOUNG CHILDREN

Chapter 1

Talking with Young Children About AIDS

Helen never expected that she would need to talk about AIDS with her students. As a third grade teacher in a small, fairly conservative town, it did not seem like a very pressing issue. Her students had never expressed any interest in the topic, and she did not think their parents would want her to teach on the matter.

The whole town was shaken when the adult son of one family, a man who had left town after high school graduation, returned with a diagnosis of AIDS. He would be living with his parents, who would help care for him and support him. There were conflicts in the community about this man—some were glad he could return for support, while others wished he had never come back.

Helen began to see these conflicts played out among the students at her school. She saw some children become anxious about "catching" AIDS, others repeat cruel or crude jokes, and many share misinformation among themselves. She joined a few teachers who suggested developing classroom lessons addressing these issues. Controversy flamed again, with some townspeople supporting the idea and others vociferously against it.

"Ultimately, of course, it was the children who suffered," she told us. "We never thought our town would be touched by this epidemic, so we

didn't prepare ourselves well. By the time we did address the issue, we were in a crisis. There was no time to educate parents and teachers, to help them better understand the need to teach their children about AIDS. The children were totally confused by the different things they heard from one another and their parents."

❧ ❧ ❧

AIDS brings up many difficult issues—life and death, illness and disability, injection drug use, human sexuality and homosexuality. Many adults find it uncomfortable to discuss these topics among themselves. It is understandable that one might wonder why anyone would want to bring up such sophisticated material with young children. It is our purpose to explain that there *are* important reasons to talk with young children about AIDS and HIV, and to share some suggestions for just how to do this.

One thing we want to make immediately clear is that we are not suggesting children be presented material that is beyond their understanding. We believe children deserve good and appropriate answers to their questions, and many *do* have questions about AIDS. However, "AIDS education" for many young children will not need to be explicit or even very specific, and in most instances it will really have more to do with health and communicable diseases generally than with HIV particularly. By laying a careful foundation of understanding, we can prepare young children for more sophisticated explanations of HIV and other health issues in later years.

HIV is an important part of American life. Internationally, it is a major health problem. The ultimate effects of this epidemic on our social system, our global economic system, our world health system, and our individual lives are difficult to imagine. An issue as big as HIV will touch the awareness of children of all ages, whether or not they are told about it directly by their parents or teachers. On television and the radio, in conversations of adults around them, in playground interactions with peers and with older children, in the newspaper as they begin to read—children hear about HIV.

And since they hear about it, children also have questions about HIV. This is only natural. Children are fascinated by the world around them. They might wonder why it turns dark at night, how a television works, or why they bleed if they cut themselves. As children grow, they discover that accurate answers to questions can sometimes make their lives more familiar, more exciting and more comfortable. Now that HIV is a part of our world, we find that even very young children are beginning to ask questions about the disease.

In the same way that it is natural for children to ask questions, adults who care for them—their parents, teachers, health care providers and other caretakers—want to give them accurate and age-appropriate answers. With a topic like HIV, this wish to teach children about the world is complicated by the difficulty of the subject. Just what is an "age-appropriate" response to a young child's questions about HIV? When, if ever, should adults initiate a discussion on the topic? What do children want to know, and what do they need to know?

This book has been written to help parents, teachers and others who spend time with children develop answers to these questions. The recommendations we make are based on our personal experiences with children, and interviews with parents and professionals who work with children. There are few absolutes in this matter—each child and each community are different, and what is useful in one place may not be in another. We hope the suggestions in this book can be used as a frame of reference to help parents, teachers and other caretakers answer children's questions.

We want to emphasize the importance of the phrase "age-appropriate material." Often when we talk about providing HIV education to young children, people assume this to mean that we want to present six year olds with explicit information about sex. This is not what we recommend. Appropriate material for a six year old would include some basic concepts about health and communicable diseases (they exist, some are easy to get, some are hard to get). This information should be presented in the context of a comprehensive school health program, and taught by the regular classroom teacher. HIV might not be mentioned at all, or might be referred to only in passing. If a child this young is bringing up explicit questions about vaginal, oral or anal sex, one would want to consider carefully the possibility that this child, or one of his or her friends, was being sexually molested. Most six year olds neither need nor want graphic descriptions of adult sexual activities.

We also acknowledge the limitations of this book. It is not a comprehensive guide to teaching children about health and sexuality; it is not a comprehensive source of information about HIV and AIDS; it does not provide a comprehensive description of child development. We summarize each of these topics and relate them to our subject, but for thorough background in any of these areas, we refer you to one of the resources listed in Section 3 of this book.

Why Do Young Children Need to Know About AIDS and HIV?

There are a number of good reasons to learn to talk to young children about HIV. Some apply to all children and some to only a few, but together we think they create a compelling rationale. We list our reasons below.

1. The natural curiosity of children.

As we already mentioned, children are naturally curious about the world around them. HIV is now, tragically, an undeniable part of that world. Young children will and do have questions about HIV.

This curiosity is a natural and delightful quality of children. Responding in a positive and appropriate way to their questions encourages healthy and vigorous development of their cognitive, social and emotional skills. In this sense, HIV is no different from all the other subjects that fascinate a child.

If we neglect or refuse to answer these questions, we frustrate a child's wish to know about the world. He or she may begin to feel less interested and less motivated to learn, or may feel ashamed or guilty about being curious. When our reticence to respond extends only to certain topics—like HIV, or sex, or death, or a family member's obvious but unaddressed trouble with alcohol—the child usually learns to avoid these areas of questioning. He or she will seek answers from other sources. The information may be inaccurate, and it may endorse values inconsistent with those of the parents.

2. The anxiety children may have about the disease.

Children understand that AIDS is a very serious disease. They usually do not understand the concept "not casually transmitted." They have caught colds and chicken pox easily in the past. What can protect them from catching this very serious disease in the future?

In addition to their personal fears of contracting AIDS, young children may worry that parents or other family members will become ill. This concern is especially challenging when parents or other family members *are* actually at risk, or are practicing risky behaviors. Giving children tools to understand concepts about disease transmission can help lower this kind of anxiety.

3. Some children may have parents, other family or friends with AIDS or HIV infection. These children will benefit from the presence of compassion and understanding among their peers.

Children who have a family member diagnosed with AIDS or HIV infection face many personal challenges. We do not want to add the harassment or misunderstanding of peers to an already painful circumstance. When children feel secure that HIV is not casually transmitted, and when they have seen teachers and parents model humane responses to those who are ill (or who have illness in their families), they are less likely to tease or criticize someone in this situation.

4. Many communities, schools and neighborhoods will be home to HIV-infected children and adults in the future.

HIV education can lay a groundwork to help both children and parents avoid harmful or negative reactions in these instances. When communities become distraught over the presence of HIV-infected children, this is obviously a difficulty for that child and his or her family. However, the divisiveness and bitterness that have arisen in some cases hurt the greater community as well. No one is served by overly emotional responses, and we are all helped by clear and accurate information.

Comprehensive School Health Programs

HIV presents one of the biggest challenges parents and educators have ever faced—that of helping to save the lives of their children and students. Young children need help developing a conceptual framework about health and communicable disease that will lead them to a fuller understanding of HIV in later years. Much of the education they need in this light is not specific to HIV at all, but addresses broader issues of wellness and illness; understanding communicable diseases and their prevention; being familiar with common health practices that help stop the spread of disease in general; and developing the awareness that those who are ill need compassion and support from the community and good medical care from their health providers.

In a school setting, these matters most naturally fit into a comprehensive school health program. Such programs seek to promote health education that addresses the whole child—mentally, physically and socially. Planned instruction focuses on health-related topics for students in grades K-12, with increasing sophistication as the child matures. From such programs, we hope, each child will develop behaviors that enhance personal health and well-being, while avoiding behaviors that might cause disease or health problems. We want children to learn to look beyond their own personal interests and think also about the health and well-being of their family, their friends and the larger community. Finally, we want students to think about the well-being of future generations.

The HIV epidemic makes it clear as never before that comprehensive school health programs are essential to the welfare of our nation's children. Health education must equip children with fundamental concepts and personal skills to protect and enhance their own health and that of the community. These concepts and skills will not magically appear in young people at whatever age they are first given the opportunity to engage in sexual activity or drug use. The abilities to make sound decisions for one's health and well-being, to resist peer pressure, to feel positive about oneself, to refuse invitations to engage in non-healthful activities, are skills that can only be built over time, in a carefully sequenced manner that builds new understanding on previous material and includes a lot of practice.

When we start programs early—teaching young children what good hygiene is and why it is important, some of the ways diseases are passed, that different diseases are transmitted in different ways, and how to protect oneself from illness—we are building that essential foundation. In addition, we find that when such programs are in place, and particularly when they are reinforced with parent involvement (through parent review of materials, providing informational meetings for parents, parent participation in some student homework assignments, and so forth), answers to children's questions about HIV come much easier for parents, teachers and others who work with children.

Additional HIV Prevention Strategies for Young Children

In addition to the knowledge we want young children to have about health, disease, and HIV, there are two important HIV prevention strategies to consider for this age group.

1. Children face a small but real risk of infection through sexual molestation by an HIV-infected adult.

Horrible as it is to imagine, such cases have occurred. We need to do all we can to prevent any child in our care from facing similar traumas. Adults should act swiftly and aggressively to protect the child in cases of molestation. Programs that teach children skills to avoid sexual abuse should be supported. These lessons should be included within a comprehensive school health program. (See Section 3, *Further Resources*, for references on this topic.)

2. Drug use is associated with HIV infection. Within the health program, drug prevention programs should be started in early elementary grades.

The best way to prevent drug abuse is to teach drug prevention lessons early and repeat the messages over time. The best drug abuse prevention programs are a sequenced and planned part of the school's health education program. Support for these programs also promotes HIV prevention.

Keeping Parents Involved

The role of parents in educating young children about health issues is essential and cannot be overemphasized. Parents are the primary educators of children about morals and values, personal relationships, sexuality and self-esteem. What the child sees in practice in the home is what he or she learns to generalize to the rest of the world. School-based lessons in these areas are not especially useful if they do not relate to the values the child learns in the home.

This is one reason it is so important for parents to be involved in the development and/or evaluation of curricula on such topics. We believe parents should have the opportunity to review any school materials, to provide input, and to observe classes. Ideally, parents will see themselves working in partnership with the schools.

It is important that the entire school curriculum be consistent with children's cultural, religious, linguistic and ethnic background. This is particularly essential for lessons about HIV, drug use and abuse and human sexuality. In our multicultural American society, community input and parent involvement are especially important. We believe the local community will have the best understanding of how to educate children, and suggest that there be careful local review of any materials to be used in group settings with children.

Many successful lessons concerning health and personal relationships involve homework assignments during which children discuss the lessons with their parents. These discussions create an atmosphere of openness and honesty, which contributes to better learning for the student while reinforcing the values of the family. These kinds of models are appropriate for HIV education as well. We hope that parents will take an active role in educating their children and promoting good comprehensive health education programs in their community's schools.

Talking About HIV: What Do You Need to Know?

Many parents and others who care for the young wonder how to prepare themselves to talk about HIV with children. It may seem a little intimidating—there is so much information about HIV; the related issues are sensitive and complicated; it is often uncomfortable to talk about these topics; and teachers may worry that parents will be upset if they hear that these subjects have been addressed with their children.

While HIV may be a new topic, most of what it brings to light is not new. Children have always asked questions about health and illness, life and death, intimacy and sexuality. Parents and teachers already have ways they handle sensitive issues when they arise. In learning to talk with young children about HIV, we are primarily using communication and teaching skills that have been used in other circumstances before. We adapt these approaches to the particular facts about HIV.

To be comfortable with this task, you will want to have a general familiarity with the following areas, all of which are covered in this book:

1. **Child development.**

How and what do children think about health, personal relationships and sexuality? What kinds of questions will they have on these topics? This material is covered in Chapter 12: *HIV Information and Developmental Stages: What Do Children Want to Know About AIDS, When?*

2. **Basic HIV information.**

Accurate answers are based on a sound general knowledge about transmission, prevention and the course of the disease. Very sophisticated knowledge is not necessary—young children cannot understand more than the most basic information. A good basic information resource is Chapter 11: *HIV Information: Answers for Adults.*

3. **Some idea of the sorts of questions young children are asking about HIV.**

This is explored in Chapter 3: *What Are Children Asking and How Can You Answer Them?*

4. **Ideas about how to answer these questions, or otherwise bring up the topic of HIV appropriately with children.**

These concerns are covered in Chapter 3: *What Are Children Asking and How Can You Answer Them?*, Chapter 4: *When Should You Bring Up the Topic?*, Chapter 5: *Special Circumstances: When a Child, Family or Friends Are at Risk for or Infected with HIV*, and Chapter 6: *Issues for the Young Child in Foster Care.*

Four Important Values When Providing HIV Information

There are four basic values that we hope will underlie all approaches to talking with children about HIV:

1. Persons with AIDS/HIV infection, and their friends and relatives, should be considered with respect and compassion.
2. We do not want to speak in a manner that would lead children to feel badly about themselves or negatively about human sexuality and intimacy.
3. Most people, including children, have sexual feelings, and this is quite natural. However, sexual activities like intercourse are not appropriate for children.
4. Curiosity is natural and questions are healthy. We want children to ask these questions and especially encourage them to discuss their thoughts with their parents.

As you review and consider the information in this book, we hope you will remember that the most essential skills for talking about these matters with children cannot be taught in this or any other resource. Openness, expressions of love and caring, willingness to be honest and genuine—these are qualities most parents, teachers and others who care for children cultivate, and these are the qualities that will make your time with children more rewarding and your teaching of them most effective. Listening carefully to children, allowing them to complete their thoughts and questions before offering answers, and checking their understanding of the discussion will facilitate productive talks about HIV or other sensitive issues.

Chapter 2

Things to Keep in Mind

"I know you are writing a book about how to talk to young children about AIDS, and I wanted to tell you about an experience I had," our friend Ernesto said. This is what he told us:

My parents were visiting, and my five-year-old son and I were taking them on a tour of the city in the car. My boy was in the back seat and seemed totally involved in playing with a few toys he had brought along, so I assumed he wasn't listening to the grown-ups talk.

As we drove through the gay neighborhood, I commented that things had really changed there since the AIDS thing happened—there were a lot fewer people around, there was a mood of depression, and I guessed it was because so many of them had died. My son suddenly pipes up, "They died? Why did they die?"

"Oh, they caught a disease," I said. But he's the kind of kid who has a lot of questions when his curiosity gets started.

"What disease?" he asked me.

"It's called AIDS," I answered.

"How do people get it?" he asked—of course! I could tell my parents were beginning to feel uncomfortable with this. They aren't the kind of folks who ever had a lot of explicit talks with their children. So I tried to answer his questions, but I was getting nervous about what my parents were thinking, and my son kept asking harder and harder questions—

"Why did people in this neighborhood get it?" "Aren't these gay men?" "What makes them gay men?"

Finally I told him it would be better if we could discuss this later because it was a hard subject for me to explain to him. Usually I wouldn't do that, but I was so distracted by my parents' presence, I didn't feel like I was doing a very good job answering his questions anyway.

🙵 🙵 🙵

There can be few absolutes when we make suggestions about how to answer young children's questions about HIV. We give some specific examples in Chapter 3: *What Are Children Asking and How Can You Answer Them?*, and Chapter 5: *Special Circumstances: When a Child, Family or Friends Are at Risk for or Infected with HIV*, but your own approach to educating children about HIV will depend on many different things, including:

1. **Your relationship with the child.**
Is this your own child? A student in the classroom? A patient? The child of a neighbor?

2. **The particular circumstances at hand.**
Are you speaking privately with the child, or in a large group? Do you have a lot of time or are you "on your way out the door"?

3. **Your own sense of preparedness.**
Have you been surprised by a sudden question? Are you bringing up an issue you had planned to talk about?

4. **Your previous discussions with the child on this or related topics.**
Do you have a comfortable foundation for talking about this issue, or is it something new for both you and the child?

5. **The child's age and developmental level.**
What is the child capable of understanding?

6. **Any special history pertinent to the circumstances.**
Has the child just been frightened by a news broadcast? Is someone close to the child ill with HIV infection?

7. If the child is asking a question, what is the real meaning behind the question?
See The Meaning Behind the Question, p.17, for more about this.

These are a lot of variables to keep in mind! It makes this task seem so difficult. But if you look over the list once again, you will see that, in fact, these are the kinds of things adults always attend to when educating children or responding to their questions. Once again, the skills that have served parents, teachers and others well in their contact with children in the past are those that will be most useful in addressing this new issue of HIV.

Four Goals for Parents, Teachers and Caretakers

Most of us cannot keep in mind at all times all the specific suggestions and facts about discussing HIV with young children. It may be useful to remember four general goals.

1. Set a groundwork.
Parents and caretakers can set a groundwork for communicating about health, human loving, sexuality and values from a child's earliest age. Teachers and other educators can set a foundation for young children to understand health and communicable disease and, as appropriate, human sexuality (considering the child's age, school guidelines, community values and the specific circumstances).

2. Help the child.
Those who care for children can help the child develop a confident and strong sense of self and of being loved.

3. Be willing to answer questions.
Adults can demonstrate a willingness to answer children's questions about HIV as they arise. They can also explore the meaning behind the questions to try best to help the child cope with anxieties or feel that his or her concern has been addressed.

4. **Be willing to bring up the topic.**
Adults who care for children can demonstrate a willingness to bring up the issue of HIV with young children at times when it is appropriate to do so.

Teaching Children About Sexuality

We suggest that parents and, as appropriate, teachers, health providers and others working with children respond to children's natural questions about sexuality as they arise. If children are not asking these kinds of questions (about reproduction, anatomy, growth and development and sexual feelings), we hope parents will initiate conversations on these topics. It is important that a child have a basic knowledge of human sexuality to be able to understand some of the answers to his or her questions about HIV. More essentially, we want children to have a positive sense of human sexuality as a unique activity between people who care for each other in a very special way, and we want them to develop a positive and comfortable sense of their own sexuality as they grow. If they hear about sexuality first in the context of HIV, they will be associating this wonderful element of life with a frightening disease, and with death.

We discuss some of the particular interests of young children concerning health and sexuality in Chapter 12: *HIV Information and Developmental Stages: What Do Children Want to Know About AIDS, When?*, and give some examples of answers to some questions about sexuality in Chapter 3: *What Are Children Asking and How Can You Answer Them?* We hope parents wanting more guidance in this area will refer to Section 3, *Further Resources*.

Give Yourself Some Leeway!
Basic Guidelines

It might be helpful to start by setting a few ground rules for yourself. We suggest some here, and you may add others that are important to you.

1. **You do not need to know all the answers.**

   HIV is a big topic, and it touches on other challenging issues. While you will want to give children the clearest answers possible, they may ask for information you do not have. If there is some piece of information about HIV you need, you can research the answer and get back to the child. Other questions may be of a more philosophical nature ("Why are some people so mean to someone who has AIDS?"), and it is okay to admit that these things are hard for grown-ups to understand too.

2. **You can take a short time out.**

   If a child surprises you with a difficult question, you can take a moment to think about your answer. You might say something like, "That's a good question. I need to think for a moment about how I can explain some of these grown-up things in a way you can understand." Be sure you *do* answer the question as best as you can after a moment.

3. **You can make mistakes.**

   Unless you have a *lot* of experience talking about sensitive issues with young children, you will have second thoughts about some of your answers. Hindsight often reveals many new possibilities and approaches to your responses. If you have an ongoing dialogue with a child, you can give a better or more careful answer at another time. We will get more expert at this as we practice. Children are resilient enough to recover from our clumsiness if we continue our endeavors to teach them well.

The Meaning Behind the Question

Another thing to keep in mind is what a child really wants to find out when a question about HIV comes up. It may be helpful to think of different categories of HIV-related questions that arise with young children.

1. **Information-seeking and general curiosity.**

   These questions from children are fairly straightforward. The child's curiosity is stimulated in some way and there is a natural interest in finding out more. This might include questions like: "What is AIDS?" "How come gay men get

AIDS?" "How do people get AIDS?" "How did that basketball player get HIV?" You might also hear questions that are less fearful and more philosophical in nature: "Why do people die?" "Why does God let babies get AIDS?" We sense a different quality in these sorts of questions, but young children may expect factual answers to such queries as well. If we answer: "I don't really know, myself," they often believe we know answers but are withholding them for some reason. Certainly, one of the lessons we must all learn with HIV is that there is much in life we cannot well understand.

2. **Anxiety for one's own welfare.**

Many children are frightened by the things they hear about HIV. They might hear a newscast about a five year old with AIDS, and somewhere else they have heard that people die of the disease and there is no cure. They wonder if they could get it, or if they will die. A question like: "How do people get AIDS?" may fall into this category as well. Children might also ask: "Will I get AIDS?" "How do children get AIDS?" "What kind of people get AIDS?" "Are people with AIDS bad?" "Can you get AIDS from kissing?," all with the intent of discovering whether they are at risk themselves.

3. **Anxiety for the welfare of parents, siblings or other family, and friends.**

Family is tremendously important to the young child, and many children might worry about their family's risk for HIV. They hear that people get AIDS by having sex or using drugs, and perhaps they know that their parents have sex or use alcohol, marijuana and other drugs. This can be very alarming to children, and in some cases the parents may actually be engaging in HIV risk behaviors.

These kinds of questions might be quite direct: "Mommy, do you think you will get HIV?" Or, to a teacher: "Will my mother get AIDS?" Some may be more general: "Will everyone get AIDS?" "Do all grown-ups know how not to get AIDS?" "Is it easier for grown-ups to get AIDS than children?" "Is it okay for my daddy to have sex?"

4. **Solution seeking.**

By the time children are seven or eight, they often like working puzzles or solving problems. They may try to come up with solutions to the problems raised by HIV. "Could a very good doctor help someone with AIDS be healthy?" "Can we give someone with AIDS new blood to help them be better?" "If we give children with AIDS lots of grow-food, can they be strong and healthy just like me?"

5. Seeking reactions from adults.

It *is* hard to talk about AIDS, and sometimes children, sensing this, will bring the topic up to see how adults react. Children may enjoy baffling the know-it-all grown-ups in their lives with embarrassing or difficult questions. If an adult answers these sorts of questions in an honest, matter-of-fact way, children will soon lose interest in the game. Meanwhile, they may have discovered a good resource of information for a future time when they have a more serious question to ask.

6. Special psychological needs.

Some children may be unusually anxious, and AIDS can become the focus of anxiety for these children. Such a child may ask identical or similar questions about AIDS over and over again, never seeming satisfied with the answers and never absorbing the information. If such questioning is unusual in its intensity and persists over a period of time (several weeks), a consultation with a child counselor may be called for.

꽃 꽃 꽃

When children do ask questions about AIDS, remember to consider the meaning behind the question. The same words can ask many different things. If a straightforward informational response does not seem to satisfy a child, you might ask about some of his or her own thoughts on the matter to try to get a better understanding of the child's concern. Please also remember that in some instances children may be victims of sexual abuse, and that HIV information may bring up special anxieties for the abused child. Be familiar with signs and symptoms of childhood sexual abuse and how to proceed to protect a child if you have reasonable evidence that such abuse is happening. (See Chapter 13: *Signs of Child Sexual Abuse,* for more information.)

Before proceeding in this book, you may want
to look over the background material in Section 2,
especially Chapter 10: *AIDS Information: Answers for Adults*, and
Chapter 12: *AIDS Information and Developmental Stages: What
Do Children Want to Know About AIDS, When?*

Chapter 3

What Are Children Asking and How Can You Answer Them?

In this chapter we outline some suggested responses to the kinds of questions and comments children are presenting concerning HIV and related issues. These answers are based on two important premises: *first*, that the adults in the child's life, including whoever is answering the question at hand, are not at significant risk for HIV infection; and *second*, that the child is neither at risk nor infected. For young children, it is important to offer this style of straightforward, confident and direct answer whenever possible. We know that many children *do* face more ambiguous circumstances, and we must also endeavor to be honest in our answers for them. We address approaches for these children in Chapter 5: *Special Circumstances: When a Child, Family or Friends Are at Risk for or Infected with HIV*; and Chapter 6: *Issues for the Young Child in Foster Care.*

Remember the points we discussed in Chapter 2: *Things to Keep in Mind* that will influence your responses to children's questions. They include your relationship with the child, the setting you are in at the time, your own reaction to the question, and what previous discussions you have had on related topics. The child's developmental level and "the meaning behind the question" will influence your answer as well

Most children of school age, whatever their grade level, have heard of AIDS. Given the opportunity to talk about it, they express great interest in the subject.

They have many questions, and may also have a lot of misinformation about the disease.

Adults want to give children appropriate information about HIV, to increase children's understanding and diminish their fears. Toward this end, we strive to offer the clearest answers possible concerning AIDS and HIV. Usually, we try to keep our answers simple and concise. Children have brief attention spans and some limitations in how much they can comprehend. There may also be some discomfort for the adult providing the answer—"Am I violating my school's guidelines for discussing sensitive subjects?" "Can my child understand this answer?" "Is my answer correct?" "Will this child sense awkwardness in my explanations about sex?"

The tendency to want to give brief, simple answers can sometimes lead to problems in discussions of HIV with children. One of the ways children learn new things is to generalize back to things they already know. They "mix" new information in with old to make sense of it all. The mixing of information they have about AIDS, sex, drug use, and communicable diseases can lead to some interesting misunderstandings.

For example, many young children can recite "sex and drugs" as risk behaviors for AIDS. However, they may be confused about these terms in relation to HIV. Some children understand sex to be the same thing as "sleeping together," and worry about sharing beds with siblings or friends. Others associate sex with hugging, holding hands or kissing. They have been told repeatedly that germs are passed when people do not wash their hands. It follows that they might be at risk for AIDS themselves because they have held hands, hugged or been kissed by family or friends who have not washed their hands.

Children who are told that AIDS is spread through "dirty needles" can be confused about the role dirt plays in AIDS transmission. Is the AIDS virus, like other germs, found in dirt? Cigarettes are a dangerous drug, and smoking can lead to death. Are cigarettes a drug associated with AIDS, a disease which can also lead to death?

Children presented with new information will fall back on what they already know if they become confused. What they hear about AIDS is that it can kill people, that anyone can get it, and that it is passed through sex and drugs. What they already know about communicable diseases is that colds, flus and chicken pox travel easily from one person to another. It is easy to see how misunderstandings can develop. It is important to give children the full information they need about HIV.

General Things to Keep in Mind

When responding to children's questions, overall, you might think first about the child's level of sophistication concerning HIV and related issues. This is not solely a function of age, but also of maturity and previous learning. Some ten year olds may not understand the facts of human reproduction, while a five year old may be quite comfortable with and knowledgeable about this material. For many of the questions in this chapter, we cannot really say, "Here is a good answer for a five year old, while a ten year old will understand this other answer."

The responses in this chapter suggest only one of many possible good answers. These are the kind of answers a child could understand from a parent, teacher or other adult. Overall, we have tried to offer the simplest answers possible that address the question thoroughly. For example, rather than speaking of "the AIDS virus," or "HIV," we use the term "the AIDS germ." You may want to give answers that are a little more sophisticated, or build in some technical knowledge for a more mature child. Be sure he or she understands you.

We go into a fair amount of depth with a few of these answers. In many cases it will be appropriate to cover only the material in the first paragraph of the longer answers. For older or more mature children, or for a child who continues to have questions or seems dissatisfied with what is said, you can continue to explain the point.

Always check in with a child after giving an answer to see what is understood and that you have responded to the meaning of the question the child asks. You can check by saying such things as, "Does that answer your question?" "I wonder if that answer makes sense to you." "Let's see if I explained that well—can you answer the question for *me* now?"

Suggested Steps in Answering Children's Questions

When a child approaches you with a question, following this sequence may be helpful.
1. Listen carefully to the question.
2. If the meaning behind the question is not clear, or to better understand the child's sophistication on the matter, reflect the question back to the child with such comments as, "I wonder what you've heard about that," or, "Do you have any ideas about what the answer might be?"
3. Give a simple, concise answer.
4. Check back to see if the child understands your answer.
5. If the child continues to be interested in the matter, offer further information or otherwise continue the discussion.

Questions and Answers

What is AIDS?

AIDS is a very serious disease that some people get. Fortunately, it is also a very hard disease to get. You can't get it the easy way you get colds or flu. We're glad for that, because it means you and I don't have to worry about getting it!

For Older Children:

For younger children, this simple, clear and positive answer will be most useful. For older children, you may want to explain more about how AIDS is transmitted, and reinforce that as long as the child does not engage in sexual intercourse or the sharing of needles in IV drug use, there is no reason to worry about contracting AIDS.

What is HIV?

"HIV" is the name of the germ that causes AIDS.

When the AIDS germ gets into someone's body, the person has "HIV infection."

Some people with HIV feel very healthy. Some feel sick. If a person with HIV has certain kinds of illnesses, a doctor will tell the person he or she has AIDS.

How do people get AIDS? (How do people get HIV?)
Like many diseases, AIDS is caused by a germ. The AIDS germ can only live inside the body. It cannot live on the skin.

Most people have gotten AIDS by having sex (sexual intercourse) with someone else who has the germ, or by using drugs with needles and sharing needles with someone else who has that germ. These are ways the AIDS germ can move from the inside of one person's body to the inside of another person's body.

What is a germ?
A germ is a special kind of living thing that is so tiny you can't see it. It doesn't look like any of the animals or plants we can see—not like a bird or a dog or a flower. There are all different kinds of germs. Germs can live inside people's bodies. Most germs don't hurt people at all, but some germs make people sick. When you have a cold, it is caused by a kind of germ.

Sometimes we tell you to wash your hands, even when they look perfectly clean. That's because you might have germs on your hands that you can't see. Germs wash off with soap and water, and this helps you stay healthy.

For Older Children:

There are different kinds of germs, and we have different names for the different kinds. Most often, we hear about bacteria and viruses. There are other kinds too (fungi, protozoa). All of them are so small they can only be seen with a microscope.

What is sex?
1. Answer given by teacher in a classroom setting with younger children:

Usually, when people talk about sex, they are talking about "sexual intercourse." When two grown-ups feel very close to one another, they may snuggle very close and kiss. They also may decide to have sexual intercourse. They will usually take their clothes off and the man will put his penis into the woman's vagina. Sexual intercourse is something grown-ups may do, but it is not a good idea for children.

(Why isn't it good for children?)

Children's bodies have lots of growing to do. Your bodies are not ready for sexual intercourse. When your bodies are all grown up, it will be time for you to decide whether to have sexual intercourse or not.

Does AIDS Hurt?

2. Additional information for older children or where greater interest is expressed by younger children:

Sexual intercourse is also the way that babies are conceived. The man has sperm in his body. Sperm are so small, you cannot see them without a microscope. During sexual intercourse, these tiny sperm can travel out of the man's penis and into the woman's vagina. Then the sperm may move into the woman's uterus and meet an ovum (egg). If a sperm and an ovum join, a baby will start growing in the mother's uterus.

3. Answer given by a parent:

Sex is a way for grown-ups to feel good about themselves and close to someone else. Usually, when grown-ups have sex, they snuggle very close and kiss, and they might take their clothes off. There are lots of other ways people can feel good with sex. Sometimes, people have "sexual intercourse," which is when a man puts his penis into a woman's vagina.

Some children have sexual feelings, and you might too. Maybe you've touched yourself on your clitoris (or penis), and it felt good. That's a sexual feeling. People have sex in this private way of touching themselves, which is called "masturbation."

Sexual intercourse or sex with someone else is something just for grown-ups to do. It is not for children.

Note:

Parents can add further information about reproduction or other sexual activities if children express continued interest. The answer to this question will be closely tied to parents' values, and our example may not be appropriate for some parents. Because this is such an important concept to discuss with children, and because parental values are so essential in this answer, we encourage parents to plan an answer that does feel comfortable and correct for them.

What are injection drugs? (What are IV drugs?)

This is when someone puts medicine into the body by using a needle. Sometimes doctors will help sick people by giving them medicine this way. When a doctor gives someone a shot, this is an "injection medicine."

You don't have to worry about AIDS if you get a shot at the doctor's. The needle is clean. It is used only once, on one person, and then is thrown away. You cannot get AIDS or other diseases from a clean needle.

Some people use injection drugs on their own, without a doctor. They like the way the drug makes them feel. But injection drugs are very dangerous without a doctor's help. It would be better if people never used these drugs on their own. It is against the law for people to use injection drugs without a doctor's help.

What is "sharing needles"?

This is something that happens when people use injection drugs without a doctor's help. It means that one person uses a needle to take some drugs, and then another person uses that same needle.

After someone uses a needle, a little bit of blood may be left in it. This is why doctors throw needles out after using them one time. But if someone using injection drugs shares needles, some of his or her blood can get into the next user's body. The AIDS germ lives in blood. So if the first user has the AIDS germ in his or her body, it can get passed to the next user.

What is oral sex?

We've talked about how grown-ups can be sexually close in many ways. Oral sex is one way of having sex, when one person puts his or her mouth on another person's penis or vulva.

What is anal sex?

You know where your anus is—it's the place your BM's (stool, bowel movement, "poop") come out of. Some people enjoy the sexual feelings they have when they touch their anus.

Sometimes a man might put his penis into his partner's anus. These are ways of having anal sex.

How do people pass AIDS while they have sex?

Remember that AIDS is caused by a very tiny germ that you can't see or feel. When people have sex (sexual intercourse), this tiny germ can move from one

Does AIDS Hurt?

person's body to the other person's body. AIDS is different from many other diseases you know about. The germ can only get from the inside of one person's body to the inside of another person's body in a few ways. Sexual intercourse is one of those ways.

You do not need to worry about hugging, holding hands, sharing food, or using someone's cup. The AIDS germ is not passed in these ways.

For Older Children:

Older children familiar with terms like "semen" and "vaginal secretion" might like to hear a fuller explanation of this process—that the germ (virus) can live in blood, semen or vaginal secretions; semen and vaginal secretions are exchanged during some kinds of sex; and that a person could also pass the AIDS virus in this way if he or she were infected. The idea that small quantities of blood are sometimes passed during sexual contact may disturb a young child and make sex sound very frightening. This detail will best wait for a later age.

What is semen?

Semen is a liquid that comes out of a man's penis sometimes when he has sex. It carries sperm, which can join with a woman's ovum (egg) to make a baby.

What is vaginal secretion?

The inside of a woman's vagina is a warm, moist place. "Vaginal secretion" is what we call the moisture or wetness inside the vagina.

Can my dog get AIDS? He has sex with lots of other dogs.

Dogs and cats do not get AIDS, so you don't need to worry about that. Usually, animals only get animal sicknesses and people only get people sicknesses.

How do people pass AIDS using injection drugs?

When people are using injection drugs without a doctor's help, they often share the needles with other injection drug users. A little bit of blood is usually left on the needle after one person uses it. Someone who has the AIDS germ in his or her blood might use a needle and then let someone else use it. That next person might get the AIDS germ in his or her body.

Be sure to mention: You don't have to worry about this if you are seeing a doctor and have to get a shot. Doctors *always* use clean needles. A needle is used only once, on one person. Then the needle is thrown away. There is no way to get AIDS or any other disease from a clean needle.

Is it safe to be around (play with) someone with AIDS?

Yes, it's perfectly fine. You can talk to and hug someone with AIDS. You can eat together. You can watch TV together. You can do anything you would do with your other friends, and you won't catch AIDS.

When I have a cold, I am very careful not to give it to someone else. Why would someone who has the AIDS germ do anything that might give it to someone else?

Many people who have the AIDS germ don't know they have it. They can't see it or feel it, and it hasn't made them sick. They don't know that they might pass the germ to someone else.

While it's true that a few people who have the AIDS germ might be careless about other people, that's unusual. Almost everyone who knows he or she has it is very careful to protect others.

What does "gay" mean? (What does "homosexual" mean?)

A gay, or homosexual, person likes to be close to and sexual with someone of the same sex—men with men and women with women. A person who likes to be close to and sexual with someone of the other sex—women with men—is called heterosexual (or straight). Some people are bisexual, and this means they like to be close to and sexual with both men and women.

Why do gay men get AIDS?

Anyone can get AIDS if they have sex (sexual intercourse) or share needles with someone else who has the AIDS germ. Some gay men who had the AIDS germ in their body had sex with other gay men. The germ got passed on between them. Many of the people with AIDS in this country today are gay men.

In other countries, people with AIDS are mostly heterosexual men and women.

How can people be sure they don't get AIDS?

If a person doesn't have sex with anyone and doesn't use injection drugs, he or she doesn't need to worry about getting AIDS.

We can all live well without using drugs, but most grown-ups *do* want to have sex sometimes. We know ways to have sex that protect us from getting the AIDS germ.

One way is for people to use a condom for sexual intercourse. Condoms work pretty well to keep the AIDS germ from passing between people during sexual intercourse.

Another way is for someone to have sexual intercourse with only one other person. Many people who are married do this. If two people know they don't have the AIDS germ, they don't have to worry about passing it to each other.

What is a condom?

A condom is a thin piece of rubber that looks kind of like a balloon. It fits over a man's penis. When the man has sex with someone, the condom keeps his semen from getting into his partner's body. Some couples use condoms to prevent pregnancy. If semen can't get into a woman's body (uterus), she won't get pregnant. Condoms can also keep the AIDS germ from being passed from one person to another person.

Condoms get used once and then thrown away. Men don't wear them all the time—just if they want to while having sex.

What is hemophilia?

If you cut or scrape yourself, you might bleed a little bit. After a few minutes, the bleeding usually stops. That's because your body tells your blood to *clot*. That's what happens when your cut forms a scab and stops bleeding.

Hemophilia is a disease some people are born with. A person with hemophilia might not stop bleeding if he is cut or hurt because the disease keeps his blood from clotting.

Doctors help people with hemophilia by giving them special medicine. The medicine used to be made from other people's blood. (Remember that the AIDS germ can live in blood.) Some people with hemophilia got the AIDS germ in their body after taking this medicine. Now doctors know how to fix the medicine so the AIDS germ isn't in it anymore.

Be sure to mention: The medicine for hemophilia is a special kind. The medicines you sometimes take do not have any AIDS germs in them—we are sure of that!

You can't catch hemophilia from coughs or cups, the way people can get colds, or from sexual intercourse, the way people can get AIDS. Hemophilia is a disease people are born with, and if someone has it, the doctors find out about it right away. We know you don't have hemophilia because you are too old to get the disease now.

What is a blood transfusion?

A blood transfusion is when blood is taken from one person's body and put into someone else's body. **(Why would anyone want to do that?)** Sometimes if someone is hurt very badly, he or she might bleed a lot. If a person loses a lot of blood, he or she might need some more blood to get well. Other people who are healthy let doctors take a little bit of their blood. Then the doctors can put that blood into the person who needs it.

Remember, the AIDS germ can live in blood. There were times that a person with the AIDS germ donated, or gave, his or her blood to doctors to use for someone who was hurt. The person receiving the blood got the AIDS germ in his or her body.

Now doctors know how to check blood to make sure it is safe, and people who think they might have the AIDS germ no longer donate blood.

Does AIDS hurt?

Most people with AIDS feel sick a lot of the time. Some people with AIDS feel okay. AIDS hurts during the times people with AIDS feel sick.

Does HIV infection hurt?

Some people with HIV feel fine. Some people with HIV feel sick. HIV hurts when people who have it feel sick.

Can doctors make people with AIDS better?

Sometimes doctors can help people with AIDS feel better, but no one knows how to get the germs out of the body once they have gotten in. People with AIDS might get better for a while. But they will usually feel sick again later.

How long are people sick with AIDS? My colds usually last a week.

This is one of the things that makes AIDS such a serious disease. People with AIDS will probably be sick their whole lives. AIDS doesn't go away the way a cold does.

How do you know if you have AIDS?

Most people with AIDS get very sick and have to go to see their doctor or go to the hospital. The doctor will examine them and may do some tests. The exam and the tests will usually tell the doctor that the person has AIDS.

Note:

Lists of symptoms should be avoided unless a child is asking about them directly. The symptoms for AIDS—fever, coughs, tiredness, trouble breathing, etc.—are so general, talking about them might add to the anxiety of a child who almost certainly experiences such symptoms on occasion, and sees others experiencing them as well.

Do people get AIDS from being bad? (Are people with AIDS being punished for doing bad things?)

No. People get AIDS because the AIDS germ got into their body somehow. Some people get AIDS from having sex with someone who has the AIDS germ. But sex isn't bad and neither are people who have sex.

Some people get AIDS from using drugs and sharing needles with someone who has the AIDS germ. The people who do this are not bad, but it *is* bad to use drugs this way.

Do bad people get AIDS?

All kinds of people get AIDS. Getting AIDS doesn't have anything to do with whether someone is good or bad.

AIDS is caused by a germ. Germs don't know whether a person is good or bad.

Note:

This question and the previous one may express a child's anxiety about his or her own "goodness" or "badness." Answers should be very reassuring.

How do children get AIDS?

If a woman who has the AIDS germ gets pregnant and has a baby, the baby might get the AIDS germ from her. This is how most children with AIDS have gotten it.

Some children who were very sick with some other illness were given special treatments by their doctors called "blood transfusions." This means that a little blood from a healthy person is given to a sick person who needs it. The AIDS germ was in some of the blood used for transfusions, so some children who received blood have gotten AIDS. Doctors know how to check the blood now, so this shouldn't happen any more.

Some children have a disease called hemophilia, and they need a special medicine made partly from blood. Some of this medicine had the AIDS germ in it. Some of these children got AIDS this way. Doctors know how to fix the medicine now so this shouldn't happen any more.

Be sure to mention: You can see that most children, including you, have never had these things happen, so they—and you—don't need to worry about getting AIDS.

What happens to children with AIDS?

Children with AIDS are a lot like other children with serious diseases. They are often quite sick. They see doctors who help take care of them. Sometimes they have to stay in a hospital for a while. When they feel better, they can go home again.

Sometimes children with AIDS are so sick that the doctors can't make them better, and they may die.

Maybe you have heard about things that happen to children with AIDS. I wonder if you can tell me what you know.

Note:

This is usually a question stemming from a child's anxiety about the terrible things that can happen to children in general. Many children have heard news stories about ostracism, neglect or abandonment of children with AIDS and their families. Answers here should seek to lower anxiety and avoid frightening or explicit detail about such cases.

Why would a mom and dad give away their baby who has AIDS?

It is a very sad thing, but some moms and dads just aren't able to take good care of their children. Sometimes moms or dads are sick, and taking care of kids is too hard for them. When this happens, there might be someone else who can care for the children. It might be grandparents, or an aunt, or a person who does not know the family but likes to help out children like this.

I don't think that these moms and dads give away their babies because the children have AIDS. I think they just feel like they can't give their children the care they need. Then they try to find someone else who will be able to care well for the kids.

Be sure to mention: We (your parents) would never want stop taking care of you. We (they) like having children to care for very much!
Note:
This is another question that will usually be best answered by reassurances that the child asking the question has a secure place in his or her home.

I think I might get AIDS. (How do you know I won't get AIDS?)
1. Answer given by parents or caregivers:
First response: I wonder why you think you might get AIDS. *[Elicit response from child.]*

Second response: It's true that anyone *can* get AIDS, but we also know how AIDS is passed from one person to another.

Remember that people can get AIDS by sharing needles for injection drug use, or by having sexual intercourse. Are these things that you have done? *[Elicit response, which is hopefully "no."]* Are there other things that have happened that worry you? *[Elicit response, reassure.]*

Since you haven't done the kinds of things that pass AIDS, I know you don't have and can't get it.
Note:
This question usually reflects a child's anxiety, and is best handled by appropriate reassurances of the child's safety. In some cases, a child may be making reference to incidents of sexual molestation. In other instances, a child may be worried about receiving shots during a doctor's visit. Explore the child's concerns carefully and respond accordingly.

2. **Answer given by a teacher in a classroom setting:**
    There are only a few ways people can get AIDS. Remember that people can get AIDS if they share needles while using drugs, or if they have sexual intercourse with someone else who has the AIDS germ. Most children have never done these kinds of things. I don't think you will need to worry very much about getting AIDS right now.

    If any of you *do* have more questions about something you have done, or something your friends have done, you can talk with me privately.

    Note:
    Once again, the overall goal is reassurance. Teachers will not want to elicit personal data from students in a classroom setting. If references are made to specific anxieties, speak with children privately if necessary to help them understand and resolve their concerns. And, again, be familiar with appropriate responses in cases of suspected sexual abuse should the need arise.

Can I get AIDS from getting a shot at the doctor's?

No, you don't need to worry about that at all. The needles doctors and nurses use are very clean. They have never been used on anyone before. After you get your shot, the needle is thrown away. It won't be used on anyone else. This way, we know that no diseases will be passed from one person to another person because of these needles—not AIDS or anything else.

Do moms (dads) get AIDS?

Some people with AIDS are mothers. Your own mom knows about AIDS and she knows how to make sure she doesn't get it, so you don't need to worry about her.

Still worried? **(Yes.)** Why don't we get together with your mom and talk with her about this.

Note:
Be sure to follow through on this suggestion as soon as possible. The general goal is reassurance. Children may be especially concerned if their parents have recently divorced, particularly if a parent has become sexually involved with a new partner.

Does AIDS Hurt?

Will you get AIDS? (asked directly of a parent.)
I know how to keep myself from getting AIDS, and I want you to know that I'm going to take good care of myself. You don't need to worry about my getting AIDS.

How long do people with AIDS live?
(Does everybody with AIDS die?)
One of the reasons AIDS is such a serious disease is that people do die from it. It's a little different for everyone who has AIDS. Some people with AIDS live only a few weeks or months. Some have had the disease many years and are still okay.

This means we don't know how long someone with AIDS might live. We certainly hope that doctors can find medicines to help people with AIDS live longer and healthier lives.

For Older Children:
A more frank discussion with a mature child seven years or older might be appropriate, but usually the grim details of AIDS mortality are not helpful for young children.

Why does God let people get AIDS?
Why doesn't he show doctors how to cure people with AIDS?
There are many things we don't understand in this world, and this is one of them. It is very hard to see people suffer. I think we can make our own lives better by doing all we can to help people who are suffering, and by trying not to make anyone unhappy.

How can people have babies now?
If they have sex, they will get AIDS and die.
Some people have gotten AIDS by having sex with a partner who has the AIDS germ. But if two people want to have a baby and neither of them has the AIDS germ, they can't get AIDS from one another.

Most people in the world *don't* have the AIDS germ, so lots of people can have babies safely.

Will everyone in the world get AIDS and die?

No. Most people do not have the AIDS germ. As long as people know how to keep themselves from getting AIDS (don't use injection drugs, and don't have sexual intercourse with someone who has the AIDS germ), they won't get it. I'm going to be sure I don't get AIDS. What about you? See, most people will never get AIDS.

What happens when you die?

First response: What do you think happens? *[Elicit response from child.]*

Second response: When a person dies, the things that made him or her alive stop happening. He or she doesn't breathe any more, and blood stops flowing in his or her body. He or she doesn't talk or laugh or cry or move. His or her life is over.

We don't know exactly what happens then. People have different ideas about this.

Note:

In public classroom settings, teachers will want to avoid speaking personally about spiritual beliefs. In religious schools or personal talks with children, it may be appropriate to explore these ideas in greater depth. Certainly, parents can speak forthrightly with their children about their personal spiritual beliefs. Be honest with children about such matters. Don't make up things for children that you don't believe yourself. Don't tell children that dying is "like going to sleep, except you never wake up." This may lead them to greater anxieties about death and serious trouble with sleep.

This is an example of the way one parent we know described death to her seven year old:

"I believe when someone dies, the person's soul—an invisible part of him or her that feels feelings and cares for people—goes to a special place. Some people call this heaven. In heaven, all the things that hurt someone during life no longer hurt. I think it's a nice place to be."

What does a person with AIDS look like when he or she dies?

Most people who die of AIDS look like they have been sick for a long time. They will look the way people with other serious diseases look. They are often very thin because it has been hard for them to eat. Often, people also look calm and peaceful when they die.

I don't want to eat dinner at this table.
Does anybody here have AIDS?

Let's remember some of the things we've talked about concerning AIDS. You remember how people can get AIDS—they share needles in injection drug use or have sexual intercourse with someone else who has the AIDS germ.

We're certainly not going to use injection drugs or have sexual intercourse at this table! None of us need to worry about getting AIDS here.

Note:

Many children will bring up comments like this about AIDS. They may be genuinely concerned about their risks, and if this is your sense of the situation, a careful explanation is called for. Often, however, this is more an attention-getting device or a general expression of anxiety about AIDS. Careful explanations that don't make a big deal out of things are still probably the most useful response. If comments involve harassment—"AIDS cooties! AIDS cooties!"— we think firm intervention and limit setting is called for. Children should not be encouraged to use AIDS concerns as a way to harass others. We give a further example of this sort of circumstance in Chapter 8: Trouble-Shooting: Anticipating Problems That Might Come Up in Discussing AIDS with Young Children.

Chapter 4

When Should You Bring Up the Topic?

Earlier in this book, we have suggested that parents and other adults respond to children's questions about AIDS in a straightforward, honest manner. Some children, however, will not ask any questions. It will also be helpful for adults to ask children questions, to see what they know and to invite them to talk about AIDS.

Children are sensitive and intelligent. They can often sense the discomfort adults feel if topics like sex, death, or AIDS are raised. Out of kindness, or because it makes them uncomfortable too, children may avoid asking some of their important questions. By bringing up the topic in a matter-of-fact way, adults demonstrate their willingness to be approached with questions.

In many cases, these comments can be simple and brief. They do not always need to lead to a deep, "heart-to-heart" discussion. But such comments show a child that "we can talk about these kinds of things if you want to."

Usually, children of about four years and younger will not bring up the topic of AIDS themselves, nor will they have the capacity to understand it well. Except in situations where it is clear a child this young needs some help understanding something about the disease (for example, if a parent or other close relative is quite ill with HIV infection), we think adults will not need to initiate discussions about AIDS with children this age.

Adults may want to consider bringing up the topic of AIDS in a number of circumstances with children five and older. By this age, children are likely to hear about AIDS from classmates or older children in school. Much of what they hear may be incorrect or may make them anxious. Such information also may be presented in a context inconsistent with the values of parents, school, church or community.

When bringing up the topic of AIDS, your considerations will be similar to those that arise when answering questions. You will need to think about the child's age and maturity, the circumstances at the time and your relationship with the child. If you are a teacher or work in a community agency, you will want to abide by the guidelines of your organization when you initiate discussions about AIDS.

Circumstances in Which You May Want to Bring Up AIDS

General conversations about related topics: There are many interesting topics that relate in some way to HIV and AIDS. You might be talking with a child about health, sexuality, or things that frighten people. In a matter-of-fact way, you can mention AIDS in the conversation: "Yes, people are afraid of many different things. Some people are frightened about AIDS. I wonder if you ever worry about AIDS in any way."

In such talks, parents can reinforce family values concerning compassion, death, sexuality or substance abuse. Teachers and others who work with children can find opportunities to explain facts about AIDS, or reassure children that the disease is hard to get. When the child later hears about AIDS from other sources (such as schoolmates), there will be a frame of reference to help him or her assess the information shared, as well as an adult to go to with further questions.

In response to news items and current events: A child may be nearby when a news item about AIDS is broadcast on television. A parent could use this opportunity to check with the child about levels of anxiety and understanding—

"Here's another story on the news about AIDS. I wonder if you ever think about AIDS, or if you have any questions about the disease." In a short conversation, the parent can see if there *are* further questions from the child. The parent also demonstrates a willingness and openness to address AIDS and other interesting issues at any time the child wishes to do so.

News stories and schoolyard conversations may bring up HIV or AIDS repeatedly if a celebrity is diagnosed with the illness. In 1991, Magic Johnson's disclosure that he was HIV-positive led to daily reports on television news, sports channels and radio call-in shows. Commentators remarked on the situation during broadcast sporting events. Magazines and newspapers featured Magic Johnson's story, described controversies about HIV-antibody testing for athletes and discussed the possibilities of athletes becoming infected with HIV during games. It was a rare child who did not hear something about AIDS in those furious few days.

In situations like this, it is especially important to check in with children about their understanding of the events. The television programs were broadcast during family viewing hours when children were likely to be watching, but the stories and commentaries were designed for adults. Many children were left wondering what it was all about.

In response to children's discussions with playmates: Adults may overhear children talking with playmates about any number of topics. If a child is talking about AIDS, listen carefully to the information and to the tenor of the conversation. Does the child seem anxious or afraid? Is the information factual, or are there troublesome inaccuracies? When children simply discuss AIDS in the course of their day, it is of no special concern. Where there is anxiety or significant misinformation, however, an adult will probably want to bring this up with the child at that time or soon after. Your first goal will be to lower a child's anxiety. Clarifying misinformation can also be helpful.

Children with family or friends with HIV: Some children have parents, family members or friends who are known to be HIV-infected. For these children, it is important to maintain open communication about their concerns. If this person is not seriously ill, it is probably not necessary to share in-depth details with the child. However, if a child overhears parents or other adults reacting with sadness or grave concern, some follow-up may be called for. And in cases where the individual is seriously ill, children touched in some way by the event would benefit from a clear conversation with a parent or other appropriate adult.

In these discussions, we think adults should combine honesty and hopefulness as much as possible. We do not want children to feel unnecessarily burdened; neither do we want to misrepresent the situation. "Yes," you might say, "we are very concerned about John's health. AIDS, the disease he has, is quite serious. We are hoping he will stay strong until the doctors can make him feel better." If the person is in a grave and perhaps terminal decline, it would be appropriate to bring up the possibility of his or her death. Death, like sexuality, is easier to talk about with children on an ongoing basis. If a foundation has been set, the discussion will follow fairly smoothly. In these sorts of talks, remember to invite children to ask any other questions they may have.

Children who believe parents or friends are at risk: In other cases, some children may worry that family or friends have a risk for HIV infection. This can raise tremendous concern for the child. If a caretaking adult hears a child express such a belief, it would be appropriate to explore the child's worries further. "I wonder why you think your older brother might get AIDS?" Listen carefully to the answer. Does the child have incorrect information about HIV transmission? Is there a real risk? Or, as is often the case, is it difficult to determine from the child's answer?

An answer like "People get AIDS from using drugs and my brother uses drugs" is ambiguous. What kind of drugs is the brother using? How real is the risk? Is he using prescription medications? An over-the-counter cold remedy? Recreational drugs which might be used in association with unsafe sexual activities? Injection drugs where needles might be shared?

It is important for children to see that the adults (and other older role models) around them take good care of themselves. This not only models self-care and self-esteem for the child, but it also reassures the child that the important grown-ups in his or her life have a commitment to stay healthy so they can continue to provide care. The young child's physical survival depends on the presence of parents or other caretaking adults, so a threat to someone close is a threat to the child himself or herself.

In these instances, we hope we can confidently assure the child that the individual *does* know about HIV and how to prevent transmission, and will act to protect himself or herself. In some families, it might be possible to have an open discussion with the brother (or friend or uncle or whomever) and actually demonstrate to the child that this person *has* been educated. One can also help the child understand important distinctions about HIV transmission—on the one hand, sharing needles in drug use specifically provides the virus an opportunity to infect someone, and intercourse with an infected person poses a risk; and, on the other hand, a mutually monogamous sexual relationship between two uninfected people poses no risk.

The more challenging circumstance arises when a child perceives a risk to someone and it seems the perception may be accurate. Some grown-ups do not take care of themselves, and they do engage in behaviors that put them at risk for HIV infection. This is not a situation that can be resolved for the child through "education." The conflict for a child in such circumstances is not about AIDS, per se, but about caring for someone who does not care well for him or herself. Support and empathy are called for, along with acknowledgment of the validity of the child's concerns, and reassurances that the child is not responsible for the situation. If intervention services (e.g., drug detoxification programs) are available to help the adult in question, using them may improve the situation. If a parent is the object of concern, family counseling may help. Individual therapy for the child might also be considered.

Children in high-incidence areas for HIV: In areas where cases of AIDS and HIV are numerous, or are growing rapidly, it may be useful to plan discussions with children about AIDS. When the community is experiencing many cases of HIV, children share in that experience. They may have friends or family members infected or at risk. They may have friends or classmates with HIV-infected relatives. They may see HIV prevention materials on public buses or billboards, or ads in the morning newspaper. It is likely that children in these communities will have questions or concerns. Bringing up the topic can help them learn to ask their questions and get helpful answers.

In these circumstances, AIDS can be discussed within the family, in the school, or in community and church programs. Children will benefit from attention to their concerns in each of these settings.

When a member of a school or other community organization is known to have HIV: Adults should certainly initiate discussions about AIDS with young children when a member of the school community (student or staff) is known to be HIV-positive. If children are participating in a community program where someone has HIV, such talks will also be helpful. Carefully planned classroom or group discussions can help children master their fears and provide support to the person affected. Chapter 9: *How to Do It Right: The School with HIV-Infected Students or Staff* discusses this situation in greater detail, and gives suggestions on how to proceed.

We discuss some of the other circumstances mentioned in this chapter later in the book. You can check Chapter 5: *Special Circumstances: When a Child, Family or Friends Are at Risk for or Infected with HIV,* Chapter 6: *Issues for the Young Child in Foster Care,* and Chapter 7: *AIDS Education in the Early Elementary Classroom.*

Chapter 5

Special Circumstances: When a Child, Family or Friends Are at Risk for or Infected with HIV

The sample answers given in Chapter 3 were based on the premise that neither the child asking questions, the child's parents, nor other important adults around him or her were at significant risk for HIV. Sadly, there are children who have parents, family or friends at risk, and there are children themselves who are at risk. In these instances, a different approach is called for.

In high incidence areas for HIV, a surprising number of children know someone with disease. One San Francisco teacher reported that one-third of his elementary students were acquainted with someone who had been diagnosed with AIDS. A teacher from a New York neighborhood with a high population of injection drug users told us that in his school, there were children in almost every class who had lost a parent to this disease. In other locales, the numbers may be less striking, but there will be many children throughout the nation who are similarly touched by the AIDS epidemic. It is important to keep this possibility in mind when we answer any child's questions about AIDS.

We believe that there are two basic guidelines to follow when talking with young children facing such situations:
1. We should never lie or be dishonest in our answers.
2. We should monitor our answers and be selective in what we say, so that we do not unnecessarily burden a child with circumstances over

which he or she has no control and for which the child may feel responsible.

It is also helpful to keep in mind that concepts of past, present and future are difficult for young children, and the distinctions between long and short periods of time are not always clear. As adults, when we hear that someone has tested positive for the HIV antibody or has been diagnosed with an HIV-related illness, we worry that the person's lifespan may be shortened. We start to think of remaining life in terms of years instead of decades, and this possible shortening of time may sadden or frighten us. If a friend is actually diagnosed with AIDS, we remember phrases we have heard, such as "the average person with AIDS lives less than two years after the time of diagnosis." Our friend may live only one or two more years. How tragic and terrible this anticipation seems!

But to a young child, two years is a very long time. A seven year old probably does not remember much in his or her life before the previous two years—this is almost like a whole lifetime. These different concepts of time become important when you talk to children about AIDS. If you say to a child, "Our friend has a serious disease, and he might die soon," the child may well expect the death to occur within moments or hours when what you have in mind is months or years.

We are also challenged by questions like, "Will my mom get AIDS?" when the child's mother is known to be HIV-infected or to have a risk. Reassurance, one of the major goals in all of our answers so far, is more difficult to offer here. Equally difficult is talking with a child known to be infected who asks, "Will I get AIDS? Will it hurt? Will I die?"

In one sense, a diagnosis of AIDS or HIV in a family member is not much different from having any other life-threatening disease. The sick person usually needs special care at times; there are visits to doctors and hospitals; nurses and other care providers may visit the house; many sad people are about; finances can become difficult; the house may smell funny; children sense greater tension among adults in the home and are scolded for making noise or asking for attention. The children may feel neglected or abandoned or jealous of the attentions the ill person receives. Routines are disrupted. In general, it is a challenging time for a family.

In some other important ways, however, HIV is a different sort of illness. Most significantly there is the issue of stigma. People are often ostracized if they are known or suspected to have HIV—some families have actually been evicted from their homes when it is learned that a member has AIDS. Children on playgrounds make jokes and tease one another about AIDS. "AIDS tag" has been played in some places (when you're "it," you have AIDS and try to pass it on to other players by touching them). There is still much fear of casual contagion among people generally.

Another concern is the special quality of hopelessness often associated with the disease. To date, there are no successful treatments and we commonly hear that AIDS is a "universally fatal disease." We are acquainted with individuals doing fairly well after six years with a diagnosis, and others who are known to have been HIV infected and asymptomatic for ten years, but such hopeful stories are rarely told. Finally, in the many families affected by HIV who also face problems of injection drug use, there are other difficulties present and few resources available for the needs of children or sick people.

Generally, when children are close to someone who has AIDS or HIV, we recommend they be given a message of concern and hope. "Yes, Helen has AIDS and we are very worried about her. But she is doing okay right now and we hope her doctors will be able to keep her feeling well and strong." A young child does not need to spend two years anticipating the death of a friend.

When a parent is ill, the child's anxiety and concern will be much greater, but our message can continue in the same vein. "Yes, Daddy is sick with HIV. He is doing all he can to keep himself strong and healthy and he has good doctors who are helping him too. Right now, things seem to be okay."

If the disease progresses and the person is obviously becoming more ill, it is appropriate to discuss this openly with the child. "Remember last Halloween, when Helen went trick-or-treating with us? She was strong then. Now it is Christmas and she doesn't seem to have much energy, does she? We are still hoping she will feel better soon, but she may not. What do you think about that?"

When a child is close to someone dealing with any life- threatening illness, it may be helpful to discuss ideas about death and dying in general, outside the context of the sick individual. This will help you establish an understanding that will be of use later if the individual does enter a terminal phase or die. The possibility of the person's death should also be discussed frankly with the child, but one must think carefully about when it will be most helpful for the child to talk about these things. Certainly if the child asks specific questions about a person's possible death, they should be answered honestly and sincerely. It is difficult to make many other generalizations about the right time to bring up the topic, but in the broadest sense our guideline is to do so at the point at which further decline seems likely and death is expected within a matter of weeks.

Often the question arises, "Should we tell our young child that her father (uncle, cousin) has AIDS or HIV? Should we actually use those words? Or can we just say that he has a very serious illness?" Often, it is not especially important that young children know what specific disease is causing their father's illness. With HIV, however, we think it is best that the words *are* spoken to the child. In most families dealing with a member who is quite ill with AIDS or HIV, these terms will be spoken in other settings—during telephone conversations with friends, during visits from nurses or family, and so forth. Therefore, it will be much better for the child to learn directly from a parent or other close family member just what is going on, rather than to overhear it in some conversation they are not supposed to be a part of. There is no question that when most children five or older hear the word "AIDS," they have some image of the disease and its meaning. Clear and open communication can help correct misunderstandings and build the sort of trust that will greatly benefit the family as the disease progresses.

When a young child is HIV-infected, we continue to believe that long anticipations of pain, disability or death are not at all helpful. If a child is asymptomatic, there is no reason to prepare him or her for times when he or she might become ill. This will only create anxiety and agitation.

Exactly what a family says to an infected child depends a great deal on that child and the particular family circumstances. This will vary for each family. We encourage parents of children who are HIV-infected to talk this over with their primary care physician and to seek support from a social worker or therapist familiar with issues of children with HIV infection or other chronic, life-threatening illnesses. Most hemophilia treatment programs have trained staff capable of helping families with hemophilic children in this situation.

We share below some case experiences that we hope shed light on some possible approaches in talking with children in these difficult situations. For more in-depth explorations of children's attitudes towards life-threatening illness, please see the *Further Resources* section.

Tinisha: Having a Mother with HIV-Related Illness

Tinisha was an eight year old who was referred to a pediatric clinic by her mother's physician. The physician told the clinic that the mother was an injection drug user currently enrolled in a methadone program and was concerned about her daughter's health. Tinisha had presented a variety of complaints, including headaches, sore throats, abdominal pain, and leg pains. She appeared at her clinic appointment accompanied by her mother, Renee.

Tinisha was a bright, energetic and confident girl, extremely social and talkative. She interacted excitedly with the clinic staff and had an insatiable curiosity about all of the equipment around her. "What is that for?" she would ask. "Can you show me how you use it?" She smiled delightedly when someone took the time to explain things to her. In a busy clinic seeing many children each day, she was a special child, remembered by all who came in contact with her.

On physical examination, she appeared robust, alert and healthy. She did not complain of any pains and was vague and unclear when asked about them.

The clinic doctor spoke with Renee in private after the exam. She explained that there appeared to be nothing wrong with the child. Renee replied, "I have had symptoms of HIV infection for the past year. Tinisha doesn't know this. I know, however, that I may have been infected with HIV long ago and I am concerned that her symptoms now mean she may also have it—perhaps she was infected by me before she was born."

The doctor reassured her that Tinisha's physical symptoms, her age and her general health all suggested that this was highly unlikely. The possibility of running an HIV antibody test was discussed—this could certainly verify the doctor's sense that Tinisha was healthy. Renee was uncertain about the test, however, and felt unable to make an immediate decision about whether she should request this. The doctor suggested she come back with Tinisha in a couple of weeks, and think about whether she felt the test was necessary.

The doctor asked Renee if she planned to discuss her medical condition with Tinisha. Renee said she felt well and did not want to burden her daughter with this information. The doctor looked forward to seeing this family further, to try to get a better sense of what sort of support might be most helpful for both mother and child.

At their appointment two weeks later, Tinisha was a transformed child. She was quiet and subdued, keeping her eyes focused on the ground. Renee was also distraught. The doctor asked how they were. "Tinisha overheard her cousin talking on the phone a few days ago, telling someone that I had AIDS," Renee answered.

The doctor was silent for a moment. Then she turned to Tinisha. "What did you hear your cousin say?"

"She said my mama was a junkie, and that she had AIDS," she answered quietly.

"What is AIDS, Tinisha?" the doctor asked softly.

"AIDS is a disease," she said, slowly and deliberately. "The doctor can't do anything about it. There are no medicines. If you get it, you die."

"And do you think your mother has AIDS?"

"I *know* she has AIDS. The kids at school saw her on TV."

"Saw her on TV?"

Renee explained, "I was on a local TV show, trying to get people to make donations to a food program for people with AIDS. I guess some of her classmates saw the show."

"Yeah. And now no one will play with me. They all say that I have AIDS. I don't have any friends. I'm not going back to school."

Renee looked shocked. "Tinisha. You didn't tell me that. I don't understand—you and I talk about everything. Why haven't you told me about this?"

"I didn't want to make you sad," Tinisha told her, starting to cry.

"Oh, sweetheart," Renee said, and her eyes filled with tears too.

"It sounds to me," the doctor said, "like the two of you need to talk about this."

Renee agreed. "But I don't know what to say to her now. I don't know where to start."

"Maybe we could do a little of the talking right now," the doctor suggested gently. "Tinisha, do you want to ask your mother any questions?"

"Yes," said Tinisha, looking directly at her mother. "Do you have AIDS?"

Renee looked nervously at the doctor, who nodded for her to answer. "Well, Tinisha, I have an illness that's sort of like AIDS. It's called HIV. Sometimes HIV isn't quite as serious as AIDS."

"Are you going to die?" Tinisha asked.

"I don't know. I hope not. You know I see the doctor now, and I'm hoping he will help me stay healthy." There was a moment of silence. "I want you to know I'm doing everything I can to stay healthy and strong."

Tinisha nodded, looking serious. "I will try to help you stay strong," she said.

"Tinisha," the doctor said, "I think one of the ways you can help your mother is by asking her questions when you have them, and by telling her about the things that happen to you at school. She wants to know about these things."

"Yes, I do," Renee agreed.

"I wonder if you'd like the name of a counselor who would be able to meet with the two of you, to help you talk about these kinds of things, or other things that might come up."

"I'm not crazy!" Tinisha said. "I don't want to see a counselor."

"No, Tinisha, I don't think you're crazy. This counselor is someone who helps people when they have sad hearts. Sometimes he can help them fix their hearts so they feel better."

Tinisha was silent.

"Would you give it a try?"

"I guess," she answered slowly.

"We both will," said Renee. "We'll both give this a try." She reached over and hugged Tinisha.

The doctor examined Tinisha, and again discovered no physical problems. In private conference with Renee, they discussed the antibody test further. Renee decided against having Tinisha tested, but she did accept a referral to a psychologist. They were invited to return if there were any further physical complaints.

Renee checked back with the doctor a few weeks after starting regular sessions with the psychologist. She felt the meetings were helping both of them, and reported that Tinisha's physical complaints seemed to be subsiding and that she was doing better with her peers at school. Renee's health remained stable and she was satisfied with how things were going.

On a longer term follow-up, six months after the first visit to the clinic, Renee's health was failing. She had been diagnosed with AIDS after developing pneumocystis pneumonia the previous month. Tinisha continued to attend school and see the psychologist regularly, and she was socializing well with her peers. Tinisha's future is uncertain—a grandmother living out of state is not interested in taking custody of her, and there are no other family members. It is not clear who will care for Tinisha when her mother is no longer able to do so.

Comment: *Tinisha's presenting symptoms were probably a psychological response to her mother's illness. Basically, they "worked"—because of Tinisha's complaints, Renee was able to ask for help for the family. The physician played an important role in perceiving what the real problem was: Tinisha needed Renee to talk to her about her illness. The doctor helped the family start addressing the issue, and made an appropriate referral where they could get further support. Both the family relationships and Tinisha's symptoms improved dramatically once these supports were in place.*

It was particularly important that this work be done with this family, and done quickly. Tinisha was able to re-establish a confident and loving relationship with her mother before the illness worsened. There were fewer "secrets" about her mother's illness, and Tinisha understood that Renee was doing everything possible to stay alive and continue to care for her. It is likely that the child's future will be difficult—she is an older child, daughter of an injection drug user, daughter of a person with AIDS. The care she receives after her mother's death will probably be through the foster system, and the harsh reality is that she may be placed in a setting unable to address her needs well. This legacy of love and understanding with her mother will be essential to her chances of future well-being.

🐸 🐸 🐸

Lucas: A Boy with AIDS

Lucas was a five-year-old boy who was diagnosed with AIDS. He contracted the disease through a blood transfusion.* He had two older brothers, ages seven

---
*Blood donated for transfusions has been screened for HIV since 1985. New cases of transfusion-related HIV are extremely rare.

and ten, and a two-year-old sister. His parents asked to meet with a counselor who had worked with the family before. They were looking for guidance and reassurance—were they saying the right things about Lucas's illness to their children?

His mother, Marilyn, explained: "All our kids have always been active and energetic. Lucas has been fairly sick now for several months, and there is quite a difference between him and his sister and brothers. They're running everywhere—all through the house—and he pretty much stays in bed or lies on the sofa in the living room. And now that his brothers will be out of school for the summer, I think we'll have a lot more activity around."

Steve, his father, said, "I know there is no easy formula here, but we're wondering if we're on the right track in what we say to the kids, and how to answer Lucas's own questions about his health."

"What sorts of things has Lucas brought up?" the counselor asked.

"The hardest," said his mother, "was this crazy day at home, all the kids were there, Steve was out working in the yard, the boys were running up and down the hall, Sharon, our girl, was in her crib crying, and I was taking a glass of water to Lucas. He looked at me and said, 'Thank you. Mom, am I going to die?'"

"What did you do?"

"I started crying. I wasn't sure if it was all right for him to see me crying, but I didn't have much choice about it. I told him I didn't know what would happen, that we all die sometime, but I didn't know when that would be for anyone. Then he said, 'But I'm sick, and I'm going to die before all of you.'"

"That must have been very hard for you."

"Yes, it was. But I kept remembering everyone saying to be honest with him, not to lie to him. And there I was crying with all this chaos around me, and I said, 'Yes, Lucas, I think you probably will die before all of us.' Then he said, 'I don't feel very good right now. I wonder if I will feel so bad when I die.' This was very difficult for me. But I told him that I thought when he died it would be easier, and that we would be with him and do everything we could so he wouldn't hurt much."

"How did he respond to that?" asked the counselor.

"He just got sleepy and said he would take a nap. Later he seemed more rested and his mood was okay. He seemed fine."

"It sounds to me like you answered him very well. I think your guideline about being honest really worked with Lucas, and by helping to reassure him you allowed him to relax and focus on other things going on in his life besides his fear of dying."

Steve nodded. "I wonder about the other kids too. I wonder if they will be afraid of dying, seeing Lucas go through this. He loves to see them, and they like visiting with him too. But he's failing now...he's getting weaker and smaller and paler. It frightens *me*. What can it be like for his brothers and sister?"

"What do they say about it?"

"Well, not much. That's just it. They don't talk about him dying; they don't talk about how horrible he looks. Maybe they don't notice. I'm wondering if I should talk with them, at least with his brothers who are older."

"I'm sure they notice he's sick," the counselor responded, "but his appearance may not have the same meaning for them as it does for you, and his dying is probably pretty vague for them right now. What about the idea of bringing up the topic with them, having a special talk about it?"

"We did that when he was first diagnosed, which was almost a year ago. It was pretty emotional for all of us, especially Marilyn and me. You think it's a good idea to try it again?"

"Yes, actually I do. But I think what you might do is go some place special with the boys, give them some attention on their own—maybe a hike somewhere, a place where you can all be together without a lot of other people distracting you. Then you can bring up Lucas's illness and ask them how they're feeling about it."

"They might not have much to say."

"That would be okay. You could talk with them about some of your feelings, and it might help them to hear you."

"I do keep wanting to tell them that I'm sorry we don't have more time together. It's so hard, with work, and then four young kids and one of them so sick. It seems like we are either working, or cooking, or cleaning, or going to the doctor's."

"Yes, I think they do need to know that. And to know you are making an effort to be with them. That will be important to them."

"I have one more question," Marilyn said. "We have a sense of our need to talk about all of this with the older boys. I am not sure if there is anything we can do or say to Sharon. She's only two. She's obviously too young to understand much that's happening, but I worry that we're setting up some terrible trauma for her by ignoring her feelings about Lucas."

"What do you think her feelings about Lucas are?"

"Oh, mostly she adores him. She loves to visit him and she likes the attention she gets from him. Sometimes when he gets tired and has to stop playing with her, she gets very angry and screams. She sees him every day, and sometimes they even nap together."

"You make sure she gets to see plenty of him."

"Yes, as much as we can."

"I'm curious about why you feel you're ignoring her feelings about Lucas."

"Well, we're trying to prepare the boys in some way for his decline. He's much weaker now than before, and I guess it seems likely he could die fairly soon. We have mentioned this possibility with them, although briefly. But I don't know any way to prepare Sharon for this loss. Is that just what happens when you're two? You love someone and then that person is gone and you get over it? It doesn't seem fair."

"No, it isn't fair. But what isn't fair about it is not so much that she can't be prepared for it, but that she will lose Lucas at all, don't you think?"

"Yes, I guess so."

"Sharon is much too young to anticipate the future or to understand Lucas's death the way we will. She will understand it, when it happens, in her own way. You can talk to your boys about Lucas. With Sharon, your 'talking' will be different, and it will consist of letting her continue to love and enjoy Lucas as long as she can, and reassuring her of your love and presence after he dies."

"I suppose I knew that, but it helps to hear it said."

The counselor told Marilyn and Steve that they were handling the difficulties of Lucas' illness well, and that their caring and concern for him and the other children were certainly coming through in their communications with them. This couple had a close relationship with one another and a commitment to their family that continued to help them through the course of their son's illness. Lucas died, at home and with all his family present, six weeks later.

Comment: Marilyn and Steve's family had many strengths. They had an excellent understanding of Lucas's condition and good ideas about how to discuss the circumstance with their children. The counselor offered some important reinforcement for them as they worked out some of these issues.

It might have been helpful if the counselor had explored what sort of support Marilyn and Steve had for themselves. They have a close marriage and certainly talk with one another. They might also benefit from the opportunity to discuss their feelings and concerns with people outside the family. Since they seemed to find the talk with the counselor useful, such support (with a pastor, more sessions with the counselor, or seeing close friends) would probably be helpful at this time in their lives.

The other children in the family might be assisted by therapeutic support, in group, individual or family settings. In some areas, there are support groups available for children who have a family member with life-threatening illness. For Lucas's siblings, especially his older brothers, there may be a need for some sort of therapy after Lucas's death as well. If the resources exist to offer such services, we think they are well worth exploring.

Jackie: Having a Father at Risk

Jackie is a six-year-old first grader. His parents are divorced. They live in the same community and share custody of their son. Hank, his father, and Maria, his mother, have a friendly relationship, and both are actively involved in Jackie's school activities. Jackie's teacher, Lucy, had met with Hank and Maria early in the school year, and during that meeting they had explained to Lucy that Hank was gay and that Jackie knew about this. They felt very strongly that any anti-gay sentiments that might come up among Jackie's peers would need to be addressed firmly by the school, and they wanted reassurances that their child would not be harassed in any way. Lucy informed them that a number of children in the school did have gay parents, and that the teachers and administrators were clear about teaching the students to welcome the many diversities in their school community and not to discriminate towards other students or their families.

Lucy was reminded of this meeting with Jackie's parents when she was on schoolyard duty one morning and heard a group of children teasing one another, "You're a fag. You're a fag. You've got AIDS!" She quickly intervened and informed the students that their behavior was unacceptable, but she noticed Jackie standing not far away watching the scene. She started to approach him after she had finished speaking with the other boys, but the recess bell rang and he ran off to his class line.

After this incident, Lucy began to notice that comments about AIDS were fairly common on the playground, and occasionally she heard remarks made in her classroom as well. She kept her eye on Jackie, and wondered if the AIDS jokes were having an effect on him—did he make any connection between his father's being gay and this topic of play and ridicule? One day she saw him with a friend during recess. The two of them were taking turns lying down on the ground and covering their heads with a jacket. She walked over to them.

"What are the two of you doing?" she asked.

"We're playing AIDS," Jackie answered.

"How do you do that?"

His friend answered, "You lie down on the ground and get sick and die. And then you get covered up with a sheet."

"How do you like it?" Lucy asked.

"We like it a lot," they both answered, and began poking and teasing each other, laughing and falling on the ground. Lucy walked on, uncertain how to respond to the boys' game. Were Jackie and his friend working through normal childhood anxieties about death, responding to the current concerns about AIDS being expressed by other students on the playground, or were they acting out some damaging drama that should be altered or stopped? Was it healthy or unhealthy? What, if anything, should she do?

In a faculty meeting the next week, Lucy brought up her concerns about AIDS "play" in the schoolyard and its potential effect on students with gay parents. Some of the teachers shared her feelings, but others believed strongly this was not of any consequence. One of the teachers suggested that they plan a school-wide educational effort about AIDS, to help clarify the students' misconceptions. The principal made it clear that schoolyard play that ridiculed or denigrated any groups—gay, ethnic, religious or anything else—was not to be tolerated, and that playground monitors should act accordingly if such activity was going on.

The meeting concluded after assigning a task force to explore approaches to classroom programs on AIDS for young children. Despite the protests from some teachers, it seemed possible that before the school year ended, the teachers would be given some guidelines for classroom discussions about AIDS. Lucy was encouraged by this, but felt that something more personal and immediate was called for in Jackie's case.

The next day, she invited Jackie to help her rearrange one of the bulletin boards in class during the lunchtime recess. She often had students come in to help her with these kinds of tasks, so her request was not unusual. Jackie excitedly agreed to come back to the class as soon as he had finished his lunch. When he arrived, he was energetic and eager to work. They pulled papers, string and cutouts down from the wall, and chose new pictures to put up. As they worked, they talked, and Lucy guided the conversation carefully.

"How are your parents doing?" she asked.

"Oh, they're fine," Jackie answered. He told her about a recent trip they had taken to the beach, where they had built an open fire and cooked hot dogs.

"Do you spend more time at your mom's house, or at your dad's?" she asked next.

"It's about the same, I guess. I spend maybe a little more at my mom's, because I have more chores to do there."

"What sorts of things do you do with your dad?"

"We go for walks. We go to movies. He has a walkie talkie at his house. Last week we went to the laundromat, and I got to put all the quarters in. It was neat."

Lucy was feeling lost. All of her carefully orchestrated questions were not helping her find out anything about Jackie's thoughts about AIDS.

"Jackie, I wonder if you ever worry that your father is sick?" she asked.

He looked startled. "Is my dad sick?"

"Oh, no," she stammered. "No, I don't think so. I just thought you might worry that he is."

"My dad is fine. He runs five miles. He is very strong."

"Yes, I know he is." She paused a moment. "Jackie...I hear a lot of kids in the school making comments about AIDS and gay people. And I know your father is gay. I just wonder if these comments bother you, or if you have any questions."

Jackie's eyes filled with tears. "I don't know why they say those things. They say that all the faggots are going to die. They say they will all get AIDS and die." He began to sob, and Lucy put her arms around him until he had calmed down a little. "Is my dad going to die?" he asked her.

"It sounds to me like you dad is just fine," she replied. "But I wonder if you have talked to him about this?"

"He hates it if the kids make comments about gay people. He gets mad. I don't want to tell him."

"You like to talk to your dad about other things?"

"Yes."

"How would it be if I give your dad a call and tell him you would like to talk to him about this? I can ask him if that will be okay. Then you can talk to him if you want."

"Do you think that would be okay?"

"Yes, I do. How does that sound?"

Jackie nodded and said, "But I have to get out to the playground now. I'll see you later."

Lucy made the call to Hank that evening and told him about her discussion with Jackie. He was interested to hear it and said he would certainly talk further with Jackie. He wanted to do so soon, and thought he would bring it up the coming weekend.

Jackie continued to be an active and charming boy. Lucy did not notice any changes in his responses to AIDS talk on the playground or his participation in AIDS "games," though she did believe his father had followed through with his plans to have the discussion with Jackie. This was the first time she had dealt with a situation quite like this, and in retrospect she felt she might have done better by calling Hank first rather than arranging the lunchtime meeting with Jackie. She also realized that she did not have any idea whether Hank was HIV-infected, though many gay men in her city were. She continued to advocate for AIDS education programs for the school. She also felt that the whole experience had sensitized her to the presence in the school of children like Jackie, whose parents might or might not be HIV-infected, and to have special consideration for the uncertainty these children might be living with either currently or at some future time.

Comment: Lucy's sensitivity to Jackie was important in this circumstance. We agree with her that a direct call to the parent might have been a better way to proceed. In fact, since she already knew that Hank and Maria were involved and supportive parents, she probably could have set up a meeting with the two of them to discuss the issue—Maria's relationship with Jackie will also be affected by his concerns about his father, and she would benefit by knowing about these events. At such a meeting, Lucy could set up further follow-up with both parents by telephone, to see whether they had spoken with Jackie. This would help her maintain her sensitivity to him.

Lucy has also shown us how powerful sincerity and caring can be for a child in Jackie's situation. We saw the difficulty this circumstance presented for her and the awkwardness she experienced in bringing up the topic. By persevering with Jackie, she was able to discover his genuine and serious concern, and help him take the steps necessary to resolve some of his worries.

Chapter 6

Issues for the Young Child in Foster Care

An injection-drug–using parent is especially challenged in his or her ability to care for children, and while most injection-drug–using mothers are very committed to their children, they are often unable to care appropriately for them. Many children whose parents are substance abusers become involved in the foster care system. In some communities, the child of a mother who is a known addict will automatically be put in foster placement.

This means that a considerable number of urban foster children have an injection-drug–using parent. Because of this possibility, we think special care may be needed when discussing AIDS with foster children. They may be confused about the different risks of injection drugs and those taken by other methods. Children a little older may know if their mother is a prostitute, and may have heard that there is some connection between prostitution and AIDS.

Children in the foster care system may be accomplished "keepers of secrets." They understand that if they suggest such activities as drug use, prostitution, or sexual molestation are taking place in the home, they risk delaying their return to their family. Foster care providers may be unaware that risk activities are being practiced, and the children themselves may be unwilling to disclose these activities as the source of their anxieties about AIDS.

To further complicate matters, foster children are often living in ambiguous circumstances, without consistent or reliable relationships with adults. They may be moved through several placements in a short period of time. Anxieties about their parents' risks for AIDS can only compound this already difficult situation.

Keeping these issues in mind, the foster parent or social service worker can speak sensitively to the child when AIDS comes up as a topic. Unless one is quite certain that a foster child's parents do *not* have a background risk for HIV infection, we think it is best to follow the guidelines outlined in Chapter 5: *Special Circumstances: When a Child, Family or Friends Are at Risk for or Infected with HIV.*

As much as possible, the foster child should be provided with a confident and predictable environment. When there is anxiety, we hope to offer reassurance and safety. If a child asks questions about a parent's risk for AIDS, we wish we could reply with a confident and positive answer. These children have often been lied to, however, and honesty on our part is absolutely essential. If the child asks, "Will my mother get AIDS?" explore these concerns: "I wonder why you think that she might." If a risk seems likely or possible for the parent, speak honestly to the child: "I don't know whether your mother will get AIDS. She sounds okay right now, and we will hope she stays that way."

If it is possible to gather some information about the parents that could confirm or deny the child's anxieties, this might clarify how to respond to such questions in the future. In many areas, however, background information on birth parents is not made available to the foster parent. Whenever we are able to honestly assuage a foster child's anxiety in this regard, we do think this is well worthwhile.

Some interesting dilemmas may arise for the health care provider working with foster care children. Some foster children are being referred for HIV antibody tests. Such tests may be administered through the wishes of the birth parents, by court order, or sometimes at the request of the foster parent. Many of these children are old enough to need information about what procedure is being done and why (usually by age three children will want some explanation of blood tests).

For children seven and younger, it will not usually be helpful to tell them they are having their blood tested for AIDS. This is likely to raise more anxiety than is necessary. A common and appropriate explanation is, "I am going to draw a little bit of blood. Then I'll run a special test on it just to make sure everything is okay and your blood is healthy." Children this age will usually be more concerned about the discomfort of the procedure than the reasons for drawing blood.

But children who are older may need some further explanation of the purpose of the test. This is something that must be evaluated on a case by case basis. When a child who is eight or nine is assessed for HIV antibody testing, there is usually something "wrong" to begin with. The child may have had some unexplained illness; the mother may have been diagnosed with HIV or AIDS; or the child may have suffered an accidental needle stick from a syringe used by someone with HIV, either for medications or illicit drug use.

In these instances, the children understand something is going on, and need an explanation.

Physicians can respond to this kind of situation the same way they would handle testing for anemia, lead or other infection. The physician might say, "I am going to draw a little of your blood so I can run a test on it. The test may help us figure out why you've been feeling sick." If the child knows HIV is involved in some way—a child who has experienced a needle stick, for example—a more direct explanation will probably be necessary.

It is also helpful to have an HIV counselor or social worker familiar with child development who can talk with older children about antibody testing. Testing can be a frightening process for a child, and a counselor is often able to provide more indepth support than a physician has time to offer.

The question of HIV antibody testing of children can be especially challenging for a parent or provider. It is essential that the parent or guardian be carefully and thoroughly counseled about the meaning of the test, and that consent for the testing is based on accurate information. When such concerns are handled sensitively and appropriately, the process will be easier on the child and more helpful for the family.

Chapter 7

AIDS Education in the Early Elementary Classroom

Kathleen Middleton, MS, CHES, Editor-in-Chief at ETR Associates, contributed substantially to the concepts and content of this chapter.

Often the question arises, "If you think elementary school teachers should be addressing AIDS with their students, what do you believe they should be saying, and in what context? How should this material be handled in classroom settings?" Our purpose in this chapter is to demonstrate some effective ways of providing relevant and appropriate AIDS education to young students.

An essential step for any school is the establishment of carefully planned, comprehensive health education, sequenced over the student's school career. Such programs help lay the groundwork, in early grades, for later understanding of HIV and HIV prevention. They provide teachers with the tools necessary to explain AIDS if the topic arises during classroom lessons. Too often, "comprehensive health" or "HIV education" is distilled into a few short lessons. Neither students nor teachers can build on this inadequate foundation to address the health issues that face students today.

Young children need help and practice to develop the kinds of concepts and skills they will utilize in later years to protect themselves from HIV, alcohol and drug use, driving dangerously, smoking, early sexual activity, and so forth. The primary purpose of health education for children to age ten is to begin to establish the necessary foundations for these concepts and skills. The school district that already has such health programs in place—including trained and qualified teachers, an articulated health curriculum, and systems by which to involve parents and other representatives of the community in planning and implementing the curriculum—is clearly in the best position to integrate AIDS education easily and appropriately into the classroom.

Specific Content About AIDS That Young Children Should Understand

The Centers for Disease Control (CDC) has established guidelines for effective school health education concerning AIDS. (Centers for Disease Control. "Guidelines for Effective School Health Education to Prevent the Spread of AIDS." *Morbidity and Mortality Weekly Report* 37: suppl no. 8-2, 1987.) These guidelines provide parameters for teachers, administrators and parents wondering what children should understand about HIV.

For early elementary grades, the CDC states that AIDS education "principally should be designed to allay excessive fears of the epidemic and of becoming infected." They suggest the following content areas be covered:

1. AIDS is a disease that is causing some adults to get very sick, but it does not commonly affect children.
2. AIDS is very hard to get. You cannot get it just by being near or touching someone who has it.
3. Scientists all over the world are working hard to find a way to stop people from getting AIDS and to cure those who have it.

In late elementary school, the CDC suggest content area that is quite a bit more detailed and includes the role of viruses in causing diseases; the existence of asymptomatic carriers for some diseases including AIDS; the methods of HIV transmission (through sexual intercourse, sharing needles, and perinatally); the severity of the disease; and the fact that it is not casually transmitted.

These are sound guidelines. But as people have had more experience talking about AIDS with young children, it seems apparent that the guidelines do not cover enough information. Children have many questions about AIDS which cannot be adequately answered by these three content areas.

The familiarity young children have with AIDS and HIV depends to some extent on their family and community experience. If many people in a community have been diagnosed with AIDS, children are likely to have heard more about it. If family members or friends have AIDS or HIV, children will be familiar with the issues. But information about HIV reaches even farther than this. Children have heard about HIV in newscasts, public service announcements and children's television programs. They have read about it in young people's magazines. It is a rare schoolchild today who does not have some questions or concerns about AIDS.

Educators working with first and second graders have been asked questions about sexual intercourse, injection drug use and condom breakage during lessons on AIDS. It is not surprising that children raise such questions in response to the things they have heard about AIDS. It is a matter of concern, however, that children do not always get straightforward answers from the adults around them.

We hope that school administrators and parents will encourage teachers to respond to children's questions about AIDS appropriately as they arise. All of these questions deserve answers, and it is best to answer children's questions at the time they are asked. Today, we must expect that children's questions about AIDS will often fall beyond the 1987 guidelines suggested by the CDC. They may also challenge the guidelines set by the school itself. If and when this does happen, it is time to evaluate whether those guidelines continue to be appropriate and relevant in the current situation.

Teachers will benefit from trainings in comprehensive health education and HIV education specifically. The quality of education will be best when teachers feel properly prepared and supported to address HIV and related issues, and when the material is properly sequenced in the comprehensive health education curriculum.

Classroom Examples: Integrating HIV Education with Other Lessons

The classroom examples included here show teachers working within a sequenced, comprehensive health curriculum. In each class described, concepts or skills that relate to HIV knowledge or prevention are being presented.

In none of these classes, however, is a specific "lesson about AIDS" being offered. AIDS is handled within the context of the normal health curriculum and, therefore, is not sensationalized or blown out of proportion. Because of their expertise, the teachers are able to handle this material appropriately so that children gain the necessary understanding; their questions are respected and responded to; and they do not leave the lessons with unnecessary anxiety or information beyond their comprehension.

A Kindergarten Class

Mrs. Thomas, a kindergarten teacher, has always felt a strong commitment to health education. She makes a particular effort to offer interesting and active lessons on health to her class. Her students respond enthusiastically—they are all very interested in being healthy, and they enjoy these activities thoroughly.

Earlier Foundation: In previous lessons, students were helped to conceptualize the definition of "germs" and to understand their role in causing disease. Mrs. Thomas had started with a simple lecture about germs and what they are. Then she used a flannel board to tell the class a story about a child with a cold who had to stay home from school. In the next lesson, she used spray bottles filled with water to show the children how sneezes and coughs could spread colds. She also demonstrated that when the bottle nozzles were covered with a tissue, the spray did not spread. These activities all contributed to students' understanding simple concepts of germs, disease transmission and prevention.

The Lesson: After the current lesson, Mrs. Thomas expects her students will be able to:
1. Demonstrate the correct method of handwashing.
2. Explain how handwashing can help prevent the spread of germs and disease.
3. List some materials especially likely to carry germs, that should not be touched.

Mrs. Thomas reviewed the material from recent health lessons with her students, reminding them that while germs may cause disease, they are so small people cannot see them. She told them that they were going to do a special activity that would help them pretend they could see germs, and teach them about how to wash away germs on their hands.

A small amount of vegetable oil was poured into the palm of each student's hand. Mrs. Thomas showed the students how to spread the oil across the palms of both hands by rubbing them together. She then shook a little ground cinnamon on their palms to represent "germs."

The students were told to try to wash the oil and cinnamon off their hands using cold water. The cold water did not wash away the oil. Then the proper method of washing hands with warm, soapy water was demonstrated. Students washed their hands and the oil and cinnamon—just like most germs—were easily washed away.

Mrs. Thomas finished up her lesson with recommendations that the children wash their hands before meals, after going to the bathroom, and after playing if they look dirty. She reminded them that most of us put our hands in and around our mouths fairly often, which is one way germs on the hands can get inside the body. She also instructed the children not to touch certain things that were especially likely to carry disease-causing germs, including animal feces; things in or around trash or garbage cans; or anyone else's blood. If a schoolmate or someone else was hurt or bleeding, the children were told to call a grown-up to help.

Comment: Mrs. Thomas's lesson made no mention of AIDS, but it did teach many ideas that are related to the conceptual foundation children must have to understand AIDS prevention when they are older. Basic principals of hygiene were reinforced. The students saw that personal efforts—in this case, hand-washing—could help protect their health and well-being. Through the earlier model of the spray bottle and the current demonstration of germs on hands, they learned that germs can be passed in different ways. In future lessons, they will learn that some kinds of germs can also enter the body through cuts in the skin. Mrs. Thomas will be helping the children differentiate separate modes of disease transmission. Her students will also gain a better understanding of their responsibility to protect others from disease by following good hygiene habits themselves.

The information about not touching blood is new in Mrs. Thomas's lesson, a section added recently because of concerns about the possibility of HIV transmission. It is important to understand that the possibility of such transmission (that is, through one child touching another child's blood) is remote. No such cases have ever occurred. Nevertheless, for both children and adults, we believe it is a good hygiene guide to avoid direct contact with other people's blood.

In some areas, injection drug users have discarded syringes in public parks near children's play areas. Where children may come across used syringes, it would also be important to explain what syringes are and emphasize that they should never be touched. If a syringe is discovered by children, a grown-up should be called to the scene.

A Second-Grade Class

Mr. Gutierrez, a second-grade teacher, is helping his students examine communicable diseases, as prescribed in the health curriculum. He has a fairly typical range of students in his class. They are not unusually sophisticated as a group, but he has a few students who seem more worldly than the others.

Earlier Foundation: Mr. Gutierrez's young students have been involved in a health program that was carefully planned and sequenced through kindergarten and first grade. Many of this year's lessons have reviewed and reinforced concepts introduced in these earlier grades. Recently, they have covered the concepts of wellness and illness, and they have discussed personal habits that promote good health. His class enjoys group learning activities, and students are active in discussions. Mr. Gutierrez often encourages students to contribute background facts to the lessons. In this manner, he can assess their understanding of previous lessons and consider their interests and needs in the current lesson.

The Lesson: Mr. Gutierrez's objectives for this lesson are that his students will be able to:
1. Define communicable disease.
2. Explain some ways that communicable diseases can be prevented.

Mr. Gutierrez introduced the lesson by explaining that the class was going to talk about diseases that can be spread from one person to another. On the bulletin board, he had put two large cut-out figures. One was labeled "Joe," the other "Susy."

"Let's do some brainstorming," Mr. Gutierrez said. His students had used brainstorm techniques before and were familiar with them. One of the rules of brainstorming is that any contribution is accepted without judgment during the session. "What are some diseases or other ways that people can feel not well?"

Several students raised their hands. Mr. Gutierrez wrote the names of the diseases on the board as children were called on. "Colds," said Stephen. "Chicken pox," said Coleta. "A broken arm," suggested Teresa. "AIDS," called out Kirby. Mr. Gutierrez stopped for a split second—he hadn't expected this one. But he knew the rules of brainstorming, so he wrote it down. "Asthma," said Jordy. "Mumps," Chris offered.

"I think that's about enough for us now," said Mr. Gutierrez. Then he took out some large paper cards and wrote each disease on a card. "C-O-L-D-S. Colds. Stephen, will you pin this up on the board, under the cut-out of 'Joe'?" He had the children put up cards for each contribution.

When they were finished, the board looked like this:

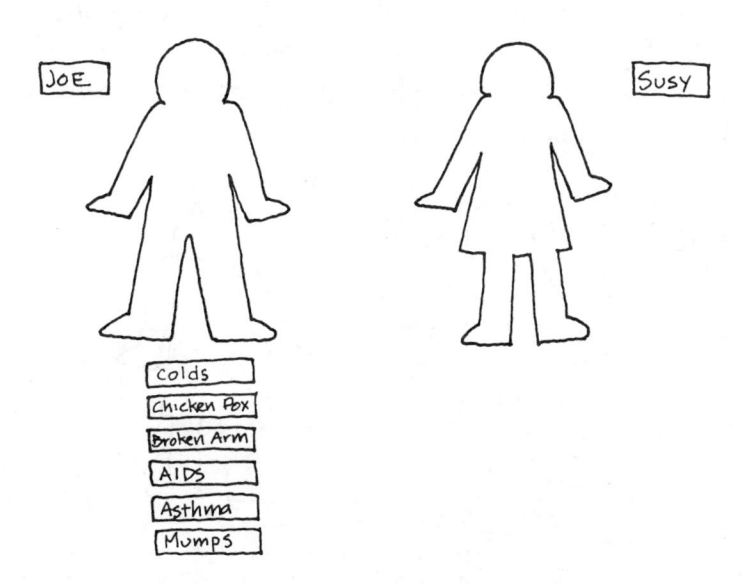

"Now here's what we're going to figure out," Mr. Gutierrez told them. "Remember how we talked about the way germs can cause illness? Well, sometimes if one person has a germ, he or she can spread that germ—and the illness—to someone else. So let's decide which of these ways of being 'not well' can be spread from one person to another."

"Okay. 'Colds'—what do you all think about colds? Can one person with a cold give it to someone else?"

"Yes!" the students all agreed.

Mr. Gutierrez asked Shara to come take a piece of bright yarn he was holding. He showed her how to pin one end on the card that said "cold" and the other underneath "Susy."

"Good. Now what about chicken pox?"

"Yes," the students answered, and another piece of yarn went up.

"And a broken arm?"

"No," the children answered.

"Okay. No yarn then, because Joe can't spread a broken arm to Susy. Now what about AIDS? Have you heard of AIDS before?"

Most of the students nodded. "Then you probably know that AIDS is a very serious disease. It's a disease mostly grown-ups get. Does anyone know if people can spread AIDS to someone else?"

The class was a little quieter on this one. "Yes," Kirby finally said. "People can spread AIDS." Two or three other students agreed.

"That's right," Mr. Gutierrez replied. Up went the yarn. When the full list was finished, the board looked like this:

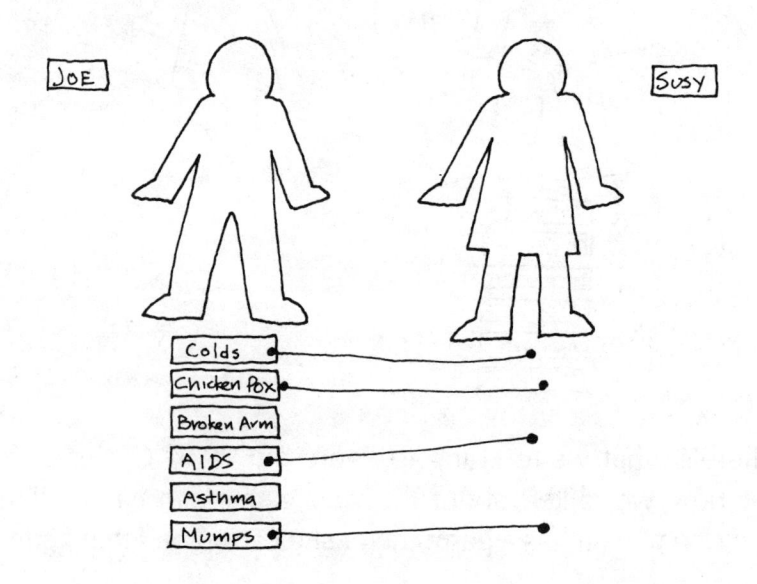

Then Mr. Gutierrez talked about the meaning of "communicable disease." He discussed the concept until he felt the children had a good understanding of it.

"One of the very important things about communicable diseases," he added, "is that if you know how they are *caused*, you can figure out how to *keep* from getting them! This is an important way for us all to stay healthy. Let's see what we can figure out from our list here."

"Who can tell us how a cold might be passed? Shara?"

"Somebody coughs on you, or you drink out of their cup."

"That's right. So how could you keep from getting Joe's cold?"

"Don't drink out of his cup?"

"Yes! Okay—why don't you take *down* that piece of yarn by the word 'cold.' You know how not to get a cold."

Mr. Gutierrez continued the lesson. The children participated willingly and enjoyed being involved. They talked about chicken pox and the broken arm. The next disease on the list was AIDS. Mr. Gutierrez didn't feel he would have brought up the topic of AIDS himself, but he believed that he had an obligation to respond to the material his students raised. He also knew he was acting within his school district's guidelines in doing so.

"So here's AIDS. Anyone know how AIDS is passed?"

"Yeah," said Stephen. "Sex and drugs."

"Yes, Stephen. If someone has the AIDS germ, and he or she has sex with someone else, that other person might get it. And if someone has the AIDS germ and takes drugs using a needle, and then shares that needle with someone else, that other person might get it." Mr. Gutierrez spoke slowly and carefully. This was more complicated than the other diseases they had discussed. "So how could someone keep from getting AIDS?"

"No drugs and no sex," said Coleta.

"Okay, Coleta. Why don't you take down that piece of yarn."

When Mr. Gutierrez finished the list with his students, he came back for a moment to AIDS. "It's important to remember that AIDS is not passed like colds or chicken pox. You can't get it from a cup. You can't get it from a cough. You can't get it from just touching someone. You can't get it from hugging, or holding hands, or sharing a bed with someone. Unless people have sex or use drugs and needles with someone who has the AIDS germ, they don't need to worry about getting AIDS.

Does AIDS Hurt?

"And I think you will all want to know that doctors and scientists all over the world are working very hard to find a way to stop people from getting AIDS, and to help people who have it.

"We should move on to our next lesson now, but if any of you have any other questions about any of the things we talked about today, you can talk to me privately later."

Comment: *Mr. Gutierrez's teaching style actively involves students in most of their lessons. He is comfortable with this approach, and his students respond well to it. There are times, however, such as with this lesson, that a student will bring up a topic that presents some difficulties. Mr. Gutierrez is accustomed to these experiences and has learned how to handle the situations by speaking simply and directly about the topics. He feels in this way he is able to minimize the possible complications, and he has not experienced further problems using this method.*

Future lessons for his class will look more carefully at the reasons that sound health habits prevent disease. He will also introduce basic concepts of the immune system to the class—that is, that in addition to health habits, which are external ways of preventing disease, the body has internal ways of preventing or repairing illness. The children will explore the concept of "the body healing itself" after cuts and scratches, colds, chicken pox and so forth.

These future lessons need not mention AIDS directly, but again the concepts will lay a foundation to help children better understand AIDS information and prevention as they mature.

Teachers of young children should prepare themselves for the possibility that a student might bring up the topic of AIDS in the classroom or other settings. While teachers should not violate school or district guidelines in presenting HIV-related material, they should be able to respond appropriately to such comments when they do arise. Mr. Gutierrez's direct and simple manner demonstrates one good way of handling a situation like this.

A Fourth-Grade Class

Ms. Kim is the teacher of a fourth-grade class. Her students come from a variety of cultural backgrounds and family structures. Several of her students live in large, extended families, while many others are in single parent homes.

Still others split their time between the homes of parents who live separately. The local neighborhood reflects this diversity of culture and family style as well, and active neighborhood organizations help build and maintain a sense of community.

Earlier Foundation: Using their own families as examples, the class has explored some of the similarities and differences among families: in the various numbers of people included, in the places that parents and grandparents were born (they cover much of the globe), in the foods prepared, in which holidays are celebrated and how. Students felt a strong underlying message of support throughout these lessons. Each family is different, and there is no one "right" kind of family.

In recent classes, Ms. Kim had read her students a story about two families whose membership changed—new people moved in, others moved away, and babies were born. Then the students participated in a project over several days in which they wrote and illustrated their own stories about an imaginary family of three members. Next the students added to their stories, each writing about an event that decreased the number in the family to two. Finally, they wrote their last chapters, which had the family increase in number to four.

The Lesson: Ms. Kim's current focus continues to be on ways that families change. At the end of this particular lesson, she expects her students to be able to explain ways that families change by increasing or decreasing in size.

Ms. Kim began the lesson with a review of the concepts they had learned about families increasing or decreasing in size. Then she led the class in a discussion. "In your own family, or in the families in your neighborhood or of your friends, what kinds of increases or decreases have you seen?"

Debra excitedly told the story of her baby brother's birth a year earlier, and how she got to be present when he was born. Some of the other students were fascinated by the details of the birth. "Was there blood?" they asked. "How did something as big as a baby come out?"

Ms. Kim was not especially surprised. She knew that this particular lesson could bring up issues about birth and death. It was placed in the health curriculum at a point after students had covered basic facts of reproduction for just this reason. She explained to the students that a woman's vagina stretches during birth, and that it is normal to have some bleeding during the process.

"Are there other ways families you know have changed?" she asked.

Ezra talked about his cousin joining the army and moving to Germany. Then Michael described his mother's remarriage, and how he now had a stepfather and a "regular" father. Ryan said his grandfather had died, which made his mom very sad. "But I didn't really know him. He lived far away, and I only saw him once, when I was a baby. I don't even remember him, so it didn't bother me. But I didn't like to see my mom so sad."

Then Jennifer raised her hand. "One of my next door neighbors has AIDS and they say he is going to die any day now."

"AIDS!" said Ezra. "Yucch."

"Oh, you'll probably get AIDS too, 'cause you live next door," said Jorge.

"I will not!" retorted Jennifer.

"Will too!"

"What does he look like?" asked JoAnn.

"Is he gay?" asked Ryan.

Ms. Kim was interested in how the students reacted to Jennifer's comment. Members of her usually cordial class were beginning to tease Jennifer and order was breaking down. "Wait a minute here," she said. "Is this the way we have discussions in this class? Everyone talking at once?" The class quieted down. "It seems like many of you have questions for Jennifer or comments to make. Let's hear them one at a time."

No one spoke.

"No more comments? That surprises me. Jennifer's brought up a very interesting topic. I wonder, Jennifer, if this man is someone you know well?"

"Oh, I know him some. But he's been sick for a long time now, so I don't see him much any more. Sometimes, I go over with my mom when she cooks a meal for him and his roommate."

"His roommate is his *boyfriend*," Justin said, tauntingly.

"No he isn't, smarty," Jennifer snapped back. "His roommate is a *woman*, and they're just real good friends. My mom told me."

"Weren't you afraid to go over to his house?" asked Claire.

"No. It's a nice house."

"But weren't you afraid you would catch it?"

"No. You can't catch AIDS by going to someone's house. My mom told me. It's not like colds or something. It's different."

"So how do people get AIDS?" asked Jorge.

"You know. Through sex or something," Jennifer answered.

"No," said Sean. "I think you get it from using drugs. That's what I heard."

"What kind of drugs?" asked Claire.

"I don't know," Sean said. "Maybe marijuana? Something like that."

Ms. Kim spoke. "It sounds like we could use a short lesson about AIDS. You will learn more about this next year, in fifth grade, but I think you are all grown-up enough to understand some very important things right now.

"First, AIDS is a very serious disease. Many people have died from it. Second, as Jennifer said, it's not easy to get it. You can't catch it like a cold."

"But I still don't understand how people get it," said Claire.

"I'll explain," Ms. Kim replied. "First, someone must have the germ that causes AIDS—it's actually a virus—in his or her body before he or she can pass it on to someone else. You probably remember this idea from your earlier grades when you studied diseases.

"Now, if this person has sexual intercourse with someone else, the virus could pass between them, and the other person could get infected. Do you all understand this?"

"Yeah," said Jorge, "but what about drugs?"

"Well, if this person with the AIDS virus used injection drugs—using a needle to take the drugs—and shared that needle with someone else, the second person could become infected. You see, the virus lives in blood. When people share needles, a little blood is usually left on the needle." Ms. Kim drew some diagrams on the board to explain this better. "When you go to the doctor or the health clinic, you don't need to worry if you're getting a shot there, because those needles are *sterile*—there are no germs on them—and they are used only once and then thrown away."

"Why would anyone have sex or shoot drugs with someone who has AIDS? They're so sick. I think that's weird," Harley commented.

"Most people who have the AIDS virus don't look or feel sick. You can't tell just by looking that someone is infected. And that person might not even know the virus is in his or her body."

"I thought that babies could get AIDS," Claire said.

Does AIDS Hurt?

"Yes, Claire. Sometimes, a woman who has the AIDS virus in her body gets pregnant. Then her baby might catch the virus from her before it is even born."

"I heard about a kid our age who had AIDS," said Ryan. "Did he have sex, or use drugs? He's only ten."

"I think this was probably a boy who had received a blood transfusion. Some blood used in transfusions was infected with the AIDS virus. Several years ago, scientists found out how to check the blood, so now it is safe to have a transfusion."

"What's a transfusion?" asked Rebecca.

"If someone is very sick or injured very badly, he or she might lose a lot of blood. Doctors can take a little blood from a healthy person and put it into the body of the sick person to help him or her heal."

The class began to grow quiet. "Oh, I see that it's about time for recess. Well, our lesson on families has been very interesting, and now we have talked a lot about AIDS too. If any of you have other questions about AIDS, either today or later on, I hope you'll ask me. Remember that you can ask your parents these questions, too."

The bell rang, right on cue. "Class dismissed," said Ms. Kim.

Comment: *Ms. Kim took advantage of a classic "teachable moment." Her class showed a significant interest in the topic of AIDS. Initially, she listened to their comments for a few minutes to get a further sense of their level of knowledge. As she explained AIDS to them, she moved gradually from one point to another, responding to the questions her students raised. The entire process was relatively easy for Ms. Kim, and clear for the children, because they had several essential concepts in place already: health and illness; communicable disease; sexual intercourse; injection drug use; and pregnancy (in discussing perinatal transmission). Future lessons in her class will discuss community well-being and how to help others. In these lessons, Ms. Kim may again raise the topic of AIDS to reinforce the need for compassion towards persons affected.*

Developing AIDS-Specific Curricula for Younger Children

Many schools have made the decision to avoid AIDS-specific curricula for younger elementary students. Because of the wider influence of HIV today, however, and the fact that schoolchildren everywhere do have questions about AIDS, we believe it is now appropriate to implement AIDS-specific lessons, even for students in early grades.

At the end of Chapter 9: *How to Do It Right: The School with HIV-Infected Students or Staff,* we give an outline for a lesson on AIDS that might be used when a member of a school community is known to have HIV. If an AIDS-specific curriculum is being developed in more general circumstances, you will want to consider developing a different lesson on AIDS. Lessons on AIDS will make most sense in the context of a sequenced comprehensive health curriculum, where concepts about health and illness, communicable disease, drug use and abuse, drug abuse prevention, human relationships and human sexuality are also addressed at age-appropriate levels.

Some content areas that might be included in an AIDS lesson for early elementary students follow. As children mature, they will be able to understand increasingly complex information about AIDS. Third and fourth graders will be capable of understanding the distinctions between HIV and AIDS. (Additional content area for children in these grades is included at the end of the list.)

- AIDS is a serious disease that makes the body unable to fight off other diseases.

- There are many different kinds of illnesses. Each different illness has its own cause, and its own treatment. (Help children differentiate between HIV and diseases transmitted through casual contact.)

- There is no cure for AIDS right now. Doctors and scientists all over the world are looking for ways to help people with AIDS.

- AIDS is caused by a kind of germ called a virus.

- The AIDS virus lives in blood and "body fluids" (certain fluids inside the body).

- A person can get AIDS only from someone else who has the virus inside his or her body.

- The AIDS virus lives inside a person's body, not on the skin. A person cannot get AIDS by touching someone else's skin. A person cannot get AIDS from hugging, eating with someone, sharing a cup, holding hands or sharing a bathroom.

- The AIDS virus passes from one person to another only in certain ways:
  - One way is when people share needles for injection drug use. When people share needles, they may be sharing blood. In that blood, the virus can move from inside one person's body to inside another person's body. (Children don't need to worry about getting shots. Doctors and nurses always use clean needles, and throw them out after using them on one person.)
  - Another way is close sexual contact (*not* hugging, kissing, sleeping in the same bed with someone).
  - If a pregnant woman has the AIDS virus, her baby might also have it when born.

- Children rarely get the AIDS virus. They don't usually do the things that pass the AIDS virus.

- It is okay to be around people with the AIDS virus.

- We should do everything we can to help people who are sick. And we should do all we can to keep ourselves healthy.

For older children (grades 3 and 4):

- The name of the virus which causes AIDS is HIV, "human immunodeficiency virus."

- People who are infected with HIV usually feel and look healthy for years after becoming infected.

- After several years (4-5 years), people with HIV usually begin to have health problems. They may feel sick some of the time. Their bodies' ability to fight disease is damaged.

- AIDS is usually diagnosed after a person has had HIV for many years (5-10 or more). When a doctor diagnoses AIDS, this is a sign that the body's ability to fight disease is seriously damaged.

Does AIDS Hurt?

Chapter 8

Trouble-Shooting: Anticipating Problems That Might Come Up in Discussing AIDS with Young Children

It is natural to worry that difficulties might arise in discussing the topic of AIDS with young children. The most common problem adults experience is their own sense of awkwardness when a child surprises them with a question and a graceful or appropriate answer does not immediately come to mind. This is a fairly easy problem to deal with—you take a breath, say, "That's a good question. Let me think about it for just a moment," and then give the best answer you can!

We mention here a few other problems that might arise, along with some suggested responses.

1. What if neighborhood children are playing with my kids, and they ask me questions about AIDS? Should I refer them back to their parents, or answer the question?

This depends on your particular neighborhood and what you believe these parents would like, but generally we recommend you do both things. First, answer the question in the most appropriate and matter-of-fact way you can (remembering the guidelines we mentioned in Chapter 2: *Things to Keep in Mind*). Then, suggest the children talk over these things with their own parents.

Finally, speak with the parents yourself and let them know the topic came up, and how you responded.

2. If students in my second grade class ask me questions about AIDS, I wonder how parents will feel about my discussing this topic with their children.

In school settings, we recommend you use the same guidelines for talking about AIDS that you would use with other sensitive topics like sexuality, drug use, death, and so forth. We hope teachers are encouraged to discuss such topics when they come up in the classroom, and that they receive training to assist them to do so skillfully and appropriately. We also believe parents should be informed about curricula being used with their children and have an opportunity to familiarize themselves with how the class is being taught if they wish.

3. What can I do in a classroom or group setting when one child has more sophisticated knowledge about AIDS or sexuality than the other students, and that child asks an explicit question requiring an answer that seems too advanced for the other kids?

One approach many teachers use is to say something along these lines: "That's a complicated question and I don't know that your classmates will be interested in taking a lot of time to answer it. Why don't you come up to my desk in the next recess break and we can talk it over." Then you can answer the question privately with the student. You may also want to refer the child to his or her parents for further discussion of the issue. In some schools, a school counselor is also available to speak with children who have sensitive questions.

4. What can I do in a classroom setting when a child asks a question, and sharing the answer clearly violates the guidelines of our school concerning discussions of sexuality in classrooms?

You can be forthright in explaining why your response is limited. "In this school, we have rules about what we can talk about in classrooms. One of those rules says we cannot talk about certain sexual matters. This question you raise is a good one, but because of these rules, I'm not able to give you the answer. I'd like to suggest you ask your parents this same question—I think they will have a good answer for you."

Another alternative acceptable in some schools is to discuss the answer with the child privately. You could use the same sort of approach suggested in question three, or you could say, "This is not something I am allowed to discuss in front of the entire classroom, but if you would like to meet with me during the recess, we could talk about it privately." We would still recommend referring the child to his or her parents as well.

Finally, if you are able to contact the parents and explain these events, they may appreciate being forewarned of the child's interest and be able to better prepare their own answers.

It might also be a good idea to keep your administration, advisory committees, and so forth, advised of the kinds of questions your students are asking. If such questions are common, it may help justify efforts to expand the range of topics that *can* be discussed in a classroom.

5. We have had experiences with students who seem to have a lot more sexual information—and misinformation—than most children their age, and eagerly share this with other students. I wonder what we should do if something similar happens concerning AIDS—if we have a child who talks about it a lot with other children, is not always accurate in what he or she says, and maybe raises a lot of anxiety for the others.

We have to be realistic about the fact that children are *constantly* sharing information with one another about all kinds of things, and much of it is inaccurate. We cannot stop this from happening, nor would we want to—it is developmentally appropriate that they do such things. It is also another *good* reason for us to provide accurate information in the classroom itself, whether that be about HIV, sexuality, or any other topic.

This becomes more of a problem, however, if a particular child is causing difficulties with others because of his or her behavior. If other children are upset or anxious because of what is happening, some adult intervention is probably called for. If the child's behavior seems out of character and extreme, other events may be going on in his or her life related to the problems. You might consider such actions as having a private talk with the child, setting up a parent conference, or referring the child to a school counselor.

When the disruptive behavior is of a particularly sexualized nature (touching other children's genitals, mimicking sexual postures with other children, and so forth), you would certainly need to consider the possibility that the child is being sexually abused. Such cases should be discussed with local Child Protective Services or a professional child counselor familiar with issues of child sexual abuse.

6. What can I do if one of my young students (or my own child) seems to be obsessed with AIDS, or repeatedly asks a question and is not satisfied with the factual answers given?

There are a number of reasons why a child might behave in this fashion. It may be that he or she is especially anxious by nature, and that AIDS has simply become the focus of a more generalized anxiety. It is also possible that someone close to the child is diagnosed with or at risk for AIDS, and these questions represent the child's attempt to understand an event of major proportions in his or her life. A child may also fear being at personal risk for some reason. Our greatest concern in this instance would be the possibility that the child is being sexually abused.

Whenever a child seems very focused on AIDS for some time—a few weeks or more—caretaking adults will need a better understanding of what is going on. A teacher or parent may want to speak with the child individually to try to discover more about the child's anxieties. An evaluation by an experienced child therapist is called for if the problems do not resolve in short order.

7. Some of the children in my after-school recreation club were making derogatory comments about people with AIDS. How do you suggest I handle this?

This behavior is not unusual. We know that children will make jokes about people they perceive to be different from them. This may include racial and religious slurs, ridicule of the elderly and disabled, crudities about homosexuals, or harassment of schoolmates who are being scapegoated for one reason or another. When children make such comments in the presence of adults, we believe strongly that firm limits are called for— "These kind of remarks are not acceptable when you are participating as a member of this club. You may not say that here." It may also be useful to discuss the issue further with the children. Do they understand what AIDS is? Do they have questions about it? and so forth.

We understand that many children will continue to engage in such behaviors. However, our limits send a clear message that it is unacceptable to do so in public settings or polite company. We demonstrate our belief that all people deserve respect. We set a standard of tolerance and compassion for others that can be emulated by young children as they mature.

🙰 🙰 🙰

Other problems may arise as you discuss AIDS with young children. We repeat here a message you have read elsewhere in this book—the issues that HIV raises are not new to us. The same sound principles that have been successful in the past when dealing with difficult issues will work when you are talking about HIV as well.

Chapter 9

How to Do It Right: The School with HIV-Infected Students or Staff

We have all heard of schools and communities struggling over the issue of children with HIV. We carry images of communities alarmed, schools facing boycotts, and children hoisting placards expressing their parents' concerns about casual transmission of HIV. We hear of legal battles, lawsuits and court orders. We sense the terrible turmoil this circumstance brings to a community.

It may be surprising to learn that in a number of communities throughout the nation, schools dealing with this very issue have done so calmly, smoothly and successfully. In such places, there have been no boycotts, no court involvement and minimal alarm or protest among parents. In fact, in the best of them, the students with HIV, if they are publicly identified, are cared for, supported and defended.

It is unfortunate that press reports commonly tell only of the communities that falter in this endeavor. It is easy to get the impression that this level of controversy is inevitable. Thankfully, we now have a number of examples that show us otherwise.

We want to offer some general suggestions for elementary schools who have a known student or staff member who is HIV-infected on the campus. We will briefly review some approaches for preparing and working with the larger school community as well as with the students themselves. For references that treat this full issue in greater depth, see the *Further Resources* section.

Groundwork

If a comprehensive school health program along the lines recommended in this book is in place before a member of the school community is diagnosed with AIDS or HIV infection, the foundation for discussing the issue will already be in place. Young children will probably be familiar with the word "AIDS," and if so, they will have a sense that it is a serious disease. They will know it is not casually transmitted. If a good community program educating adults about HIV has been carried out, the children's knowledge can be reinforced at home by parents. Having this knowledge about HIV infection and confidently believing it are the most important factors for a community coping with an HIV-infected individual in a school setting.

It is important to have policies addressing these issues in place before situations arise, and to have carried out a campaign to inform parents, teachers and the larger community of what these policies are. Most policies state that, while circumstances will be judged on a case-by-case basis, the most normal and unrestricted setting possible will be advocated for an HIV-infected child, and HIV-infected staff will continue to work as long as they are physically and mentally capable of doing so. These standards are consistent with the recommendations of the Centers for Disease Control, the American Academy of Pediatrics and current trends in legal decisions. Many school districts also state explicitly in their policy guidelines that the identity of an HIV-infected student or staff member will be protected and that the names of these individuals will not be disclosed to teachers or parents.

All schools and community programs should establish infection control guidelines and ensure that staff and volunteers understand and abide by them. These guidelines help protect children and adults from a variety of infectious diseases. "Universal precautions" established by the Centers for Disease Control are the standard in infection control.

This simply means that whenever a nurse or first-aid provider (including nonmedical staff) is working in a situation where visible blood is present, direct contact with the blood should be avoided. Latex gloves should be readily available for staff and should be worn in these situations. Spills of blood or bloody body fluids should be cleaned with a 1:10 solution of household bleach (one part bleach mixed with nine parts water). Hands should be washed in soapy water when finished, as should any skin which has been exposed to blood.

These guidelines should be implemented whether or not HIV-infected individuals are known to be present in a school or organization.

If and When It Happens: Informing Teachers, Parents, Students and the Community at Large

In some large cities known to have a high incidence of HIV infection, school districts have issued statements to the effect that "it will inevitably happen that we have HIV-infected staff or students at our schools. It may have (or has) happened already. We have no intention of making announcements to the press, parents or students as such cases arise. Our policies regarding HIV-infected students are on record, and may be examined by any interested parties."

In other settings, this approach may be less practical. While we fully expect to see HIV-infected children in New York City, New Jersey, Los Angeles or San Francisco, there is a greater element of surprise when this happens in some other areas. It may be more difficult to protect the identity of the affected individual in some places. If a community has only one elementary school, and one student in that school has been hospitalized with a serious, unnamed illness, and word gets out that there is an HIV-infected student attending the local elementary school, people will draw reasonable conclusions about who this child is.

Many approaches that will meet with success in this situation are possible. We would like to present the story of a hypothetical community making a series of good choices in dealing with the presence of an HIV-infected child in one of its schools. The steps we describe here are based on actual practices followed by several different communities that faced such a circumstance and had a successful experience with their students, school personnel, parents and the larger community. None of these communities did all the things we describe, but we hope our story suggests a good range of possibilities for schools or community programs that may face similar situations in the future.

Our Imaginary Community

Our imaginary community is a medium-sized one, with several elementary and middle schools and two high schools. A comprehensive K-12 school health program has been in place in the district for a number of years. Specific lessons on HIV have been taught in the middle and high schools. Simpler, HIV-specific lessons are also being offered to fifth and sixth graders. For younger children, AIDS has been presented as an integrated part of topics such as illness and wellness, community health, disease prevention and so forth.

Community education on HIV has also been provided by the local health department. They have offered education at a number of events including community club meetings, the county fair, special forums for businesses, citywide health fairs, local health clinics, and through the adult education program at the community college. Physicians in private practice have also been invited to trainings and may subscribe to a free quarterly newsletter addressing issues of HIV information and treatment.

Policies concerning school attendance by HIV-infected students were put in place some years ago. These policies support the full participation of any such student in school activities as long as such participation is appropriate for the child. Parents and the larger community have been informed of the school district's policies.

What Happened

A principal at one of the elementary schools was informed by parents of one of her students that their son had been diagnosed with AIDS. The principal discussed the situation with the parents at some length, reviewing the possible courses of action. Most importantly, she asked them whether they felt some steps should be taken to inform the community about their son's circumstances. The parents wanted their family to feel comfortable discussing this matter with friends, and did not want to feel they had to maintain secrecy about something affecting them as deeply as their son's AIDS diagnosis. They also trusted that the school and the community could handle this situation well, which is why they had come to the principal in the first place.

The principal and parents then reviewed an outline that had been developed by an HIV task force two years earlier. It involved a broad plan to inform schools and the larger community that an unnamed student at one of the schools had been found to have HIV. With a few minor adjustments, the plan seemed sound and appropriate for this family and this community. Principal and parents agreed to proceed.

Next the principal informed the superintendent of the situation. The superintendent assembled a special, closed meeting of the school board to discuss the issue. The parents' wishes were shared with the board and the board members set about implementing the plan of the HIV task force. An informational packet was assembled that included a cover letter from the superintendent explaining the situation, information about HIV transmission, and a summary of the school district's policies concerning students with infectious diseases.

A meeting was held with a small group of teachers who were informed of the circumstances and asked to review the materials in the information packet. A local physician knowledgeable about HIV also spoke with the teachers, answering their questions and responding to their concerns. The packet and the discussion were evaluated by the teachers: Did they find the materials helpful? Did their questions seem adequately addressed? Was their physician speaker credible and reassuring?

The response was positive, so the packet was distributed to all teachers and parents in the district, along with an invitation to attend an informational session on HIV for parents, set for an evening the following week. An upcoming date was selected on which students in the district would be taught a special class on HIV, and parents were notified of these planned sessions as well. It was suggested that they might want to discuss the issue with their children before the class itself was taught, and guidelines for parent-child discussions on HIV were included in the packet.

Meanwhile, contacts with the local media had been carefully planned as well. The media agreed not to release the news until after the parent packages were sent. Their reporting was factual without being incendiary. The emphasis of news stories was on the community's concern for the family affected and their willingness to support one of their own in time of need.

Contact was also made with representatives of local independent and religious schools. The sense of community partnership continued—these schools, aware of the circumstances, set up educational sessions with their teachers and parents. There was a unified sense throughout the district that the correct course had been chosen by the public schools.

The parent meeting was well attended. The physician speaker, having been carefully evaluated by the teachers' group, was well received by the audience at the meeting. The superintendent also spoke, focusing especially on the role of the community, their need to support this family in distress, and their opportunity to teach their children some important lessons about family, loyalty and community. The audience was divided into small groups to discuss personal concerns, and they were led in exercises to help them prepare to talk about HIV with their children.

Local religious leaders were also contacted. They were, of course, well aware of the circumstances since they had read about this in the newspaper, and some of them were also parents of district students. The school district invited their collaboration in this effort to inform and strengthen the community. Many of them presented sermons stressing tolerance, compassion and the need to be well informed on the issue during the week following the parent meeting.

Teachers were also given training on how to present materials about HIV to their students. Mentor teachers helped develop special lesson plans for each school level: early elementary, later elementary, middle and high school. These plans were simple in nature and were integrated as a natural part of the normal health curriculum. Teachers acknowledged the fact that an HIV-infected student would be attending a district school and explored students' reactions to the news.

In all of this effort and discussion, the actual identity of the diagnosed child was never released. In time, the family became identified to many in the community because they, of their own choosing, informed friends and others. The community had been well educated at that point and, for the most part, the parents and their son were supported and helped by others. The task force's carefully designed plan, aimed at offering correct information and building community cohesion, was successful both at the broader community level and in the more personal realm of this family's experience.

What Was Taught to the Early Elementary Students

In our hypothetical community, the early elementary students had already been provided a conceptual foundation about healthful living and disease prevention in the normal health curriculum. They were familiar with the differences between illness and wellness. They knew that some diseases are contagious while others are not, and they knew there are ways to prevent some diseases. AIDS had been mentioned in passing in a number of the classrooms as children raised their own questions during health discussions.

Teachers of these students were given a special training so that they had a sound general background on HIV information and a sense of how to answer young children's questions about AIDS. School guidelines for discussions of sensitive topics like sexuality and drug use were reviewed. A class discussion outline, included below, was distributed and reviewed. Because children at this age do not have long attention spans, the discussion sessions were designed to last only 30 minutes or so. If classes were very interested in the topic, the teachers were encouraged to bring it up again on a later day in the week.

Class Discussion Outline

I. Review.
   Review basic information about diseases and disease prevention.
II. Introduce topic.
   "There have been some news stories and special parent meetings in our town lately concerning a student in one of our schools who is ill. Have any of you heard about this? Some of you may have talked about it with your parents. What is the illness this student has?"
III. Develop discussion.
   "Yes, it's AIDS. I wonder what kinds of things you have heard about AIDS."
IV. Answer questions.
   A. Respond to questions and concerns raised by students. (Responses can be based on the answers given in this book in Chapter 3: *What Are Children Asking and How Can You Answer Them?*)
   B. Emphasize that people are not at risk through casual contact.
V. Conclusion.
   A. No risk through casual contact.
   B. If someone is ill, we should do our best to help them and be kind to them.

C. Discuss: What are some ways we can help people who are sick?
   1. Send cards.
   2. Call on the phone.
   3. Visit.
   4. Take flowers or other gifts.
   5. Give them their favorite foods.
   6. Help with chores if a person can't do them himself or herself.
   7. Other ideas?
VI. Exercise.
   A. Students draw a picture showing a way to help out someone who is ill.
   B. Students take pictures home and discuss them with parents. Ask parents to help students write a description of their picture and what it shows.
   C. [Optional] Post pictures and descriptions in the classroom, or in other locations throughout the school or community.

The teachers of young children had a meeting after this session to discuss their own and their students' reactions to the lessons, get any necessary help or advice on difficult questions, and evaluate the success of the program. They felt for the most part that their students had been interested and concerned. Many also felt that the lessons had helped decrease any anxieties about AIDS and increase their sense of community cohesion and involvement.

❧ ❧ ❧

While we cannot guarantee that a similar course of events will always meet with success, we know that these sorts of approaches have been helpful in some communities. We hope this sense of an "ideal" setting will remind us that better outcomes are possible and worth striving for.

SECTION 2

BACKGROUND INFORMATION

Chapter 10

HIV Information: Answers for Adults

This chapter covers quite a bit of information about HIV. Reading it will give you a general understanding of the disease and the epidemic. Having this foundation of knowledge will help you determine how to best answer young children's questions about AIDS.

Much of this information is too sophisticated for young children and we are not suggesting you use these answers with them. Please see Chapter 3: *What Are Children Asking and How Can You Answer Them?* for examples of answers to children's questions.

INFORMATION FOR ADULTS

General Information

What is AIDS? What is HIV?

AIDS is a disease that breaks down a part of the body's immune system, leaving a person vulnerable to a variety of unusual, life-threatening illnesses. People with AIDS may also suffer from neurologic problems, including forgetfulness, difficulty walking and confusion.

HIV is the name of the virus that causes AIDS. "HIV" stands for "human immunodeficiency virus."

People may be infected with HIV for many years before they develop signs or symptoms of illness. An AIDS diagnosis is given when an individual with HIV infection meets certain medical criteria. Usually, this is at an advanced stage of HIV infection.

How do people get HIV?

HIV lives in certain body fluids, especially blood, semen and vaginal fluids. People become infected with HIV by taking the blood, semen or vaginal fluids of an infected person into their body. There are four ways this might happen:

1. **Unprotected sexual intercourse.** People may take in the blood, semen or vaginal fluids of a sexual partner during vaginal, oral and anal intercourse. "Unprotected" intercourse means no condom or latex barrier was used.
2. **Sharing needles or other equipment in injection drug use.** Injection drug users frequently share needles. Small amounts of blood may remain on a needle as it is passed from person to person. Sharing needles for other purposes (tattooing, ear or body piercing, injecting steroids or insulin) is also risky.
3. **From an infected woman to her fetus or newborn.** A pregnant woman with HIV has a 20 to 30 percent chance of passing the virus on to her fetus or newborn.
4. **Through an exchange of blood or other internal body fluids or tissues.** Several years ago, a number of people were infected

INFORMATION FOR ADULTS

with HIV through blood transfusions. People with hemophilia were treated with medicines manufactured from human blood, and many became infected with HIV as a result of this. Today, medicines for hemophilia are manufactured so they cannot transmit HIV, and blood donated for transfusions is tested for the presence of HIV. The risk of HIV in a blood transfusion today is very small—about 1 in 100,000.

A few cases of HIV transmission have been traced to human organ transplants—organs were transplanted from a person with HIV and the recipient later developed the disease. Screening procedures are in place now to prevent such cases.

Some health care workers have become infected with HIV through accidents in which they were stuck with infected needles or exposed to blood or internal fluids of persons with HIV. Established infection control guidelines can help prevent such accidents.

People do *not* get HIV in day-to-day, casual contact with family, friends, acquaintances, workmates or the population at large.

How can people protect themselves from HIV?

1. Do not have unprotected intercourse (vaginal, oral or anal) with anyone unless you are *certain* that person does not have HIV. If there is any doubt, use condoms or latex barriers, or avoid intercourse.
2. Never share needles or other equipment for injection drug use, ear or body piercing, tattooing or any other purpose. If you do share, clean needles and equipment with bleach before sharing.
3. Health care workers should follow universal precautions for avoiding the transmission of bloodborne diseases.

INFORMATION FOR ADULTS

Who can become infected with HIV?

Anyone can become infected with HIV if he or she has unprotected sexual intercourse or shares needles with someone else who is infected.

Are heterosexuals really at risk for HIV?

Yes. While most cases of AIDS in the United States today are diagnosed among gay men or injection drug users, the percentage of people whose only risk is heterosexual contact has grown. In 1984, for example, fewer than 1 percent of all AIDS cases were heterosexual transmission cases (about 50 people). By the end of 1991, 7 percent of all AIDS cases were heterosexual transmission cases—a total of about 12,000 individuals.

In many other countries, HIV is transmitted primarily through heterosexual contact.

The relative risk for heterosexuals in most parts of the United States today is small. Those at highest risk are people with multiple sex partners in areas where HIV is already widespread. Heterosexuals, like other people, can keep their risks small by following safer sex guidelines and not sharing needles.

Can lesbians become infected with HIV?

Yes. Lesbians can contract HIV the same way anyone else can: by taking the blood, semen or vaginal fluids of an infected person into their bodies.

Lesbians who have sex only with women might engage in unsafe sexual activities that could expose them to HIV. For example, oral sex performed on a woman with HIV is believed to carry HIV-related risks.

Some lesbians have had sexual relationships with men in the past. Some have current sexual relationships with men. Others have used donor insemination to conceive a pregnancy. If male partners in any of these instances had HIV, there would be an HIV risk for the woman.

There are also lesbians who have shared needles in injection drug use or other activities.

INFORMATION FOR ADULTS

Because few statistics are kept on lesbians with HIV, we cannot estimate how many lesbians might have HIV infection.

Are teenagers at risk for HIV?

Yes. Teenagers often experiment with drugs and sexual behavior. Some teenagers are sexually active with a number of different partners. Condom use, while increasing among teens, is still not widespread.

Because a person may have HIV for many years without being diagnosed with AIDS, the number of teenagers with AIDS is much lower than the number of teenagers with HIV.

At the end of 1991, over 8,000 teenagers and young adults (under age 25) had been diagnosed with AIDS. Most of the young adults were probably infected during their teens.

These figures make it clear that HIV prevention education for teenagers is especially important.

More Questions About Transmission

What is "safer sex"?

Safer sex involves sexual activities that carry little or no risk of exchanging blood, semen or vaginal fluids between partners.

Some safer sex activities include:
- Masturbation, alone or with a partner.
- Massage, erotic touch.
- Telephone sex (talking with someone about sex on the telephone).
- Fantasy, reading or writing erotic stories.
- Watching someone else touch themselves sexually.
- Sexual intercourse using a condom or latex barrier (some risk involved because the condom/barrier might break or slip off).

Does AIDS Hurt?

INFORMATION FOR ADULTS

If two people are confident that neither is infected with HIV, an exchange of blood, semen or vaginal fluids would not carry an HIV risk.

What relationship do alcohol and non-injection drugs have to HIV risk?

People who drink or use recreational drugs often do so because the substances help them feel more relaxed and comfortable. They may also feel "disinhibited"—they are more likely to do things under the influence of drugs or alcohol that they would not otherwise do. Additionally, alcohol and most drugs affect judgment and fine motor coordination.

A person who has made a commitment to follow safer sex guidelines, or to have a monogamous relationship with one partner, might not follow through on that commitment under the disinhibiting effects of alcohol or drugs. Also, the fine motor impairment may make it difficult to use a condom or latex barrier.

In some studies, alcohol has been the substance most commonly associated with the practice of HIV risk sexual behaviors.

Can people get HIV through oral sex?

Yes. There are several documented cases of HIV transmission through oral sex in the medical literature. Most cases reported so far have involved the swallowing of semen. However, some individuals with HIV have insisted their only risk factor was having oral sex performed on them by a person with HIV.

Vaginal fluids and menstrual blood also carry HIV. Oral sex performed on a woman infected with HIV would also be considered a risky activity.

Can people get HIV from insect bites?

No. There has never been a documented case of HIV transmission associated with insect bites, and many researchers have looked carefully for such evidence.

Epidemiologic studies (who gets HIV, how and where) throughout the world reinforce researchers' findings. Consistently, people who have HIV

INFORMATION FOR ADULTS

also have some other identifiable risk activity, such as unprotected sexual intercourse with an infected person, sharing of needles, or being born to a mother with HIV. The greater population of people bitten by insects includes large numbers of children ages six to twelve, and many elders. These individuals are rarely diagnosed with AIDS, and those who are have identifiable risks.

Household studies of thousands of people with AIDS and HIV have shown transmission within households only where identifiable risks have occurred—for example, when a man and woman have had unprotected sexual intercourse. Household members who might presumably be bitten by the same insects have not developed HIV.

Can people still get HIV from blood transfusions?

The risk of contracting HIV through a blood transfusion is extremely small—far less than the risk of serious physical harm should an individual refuse a needed transfusion.

Most people at known risk for HIV voluntarily avoid donating blood. Additionally, the HIV antibody test is performed on all blood in the United States donated for medical purposes. Estimates of the actual risk of a given unit of blood being infected range from 1 in 20,000 to about 1 in 100,000.

Blood can carry a number of different human viruses, including HIV, hepatitis-B, and other forms of hepatitis. Because of the potential for infections to be transmitted during blood transfusions, physicians today recommend transfusions only when they are absolutely necessary. For elective surgeries, people are often able to arrange to "donate" their own blood beforehand, to preclude any chance of new infections being introduced into the body.

Can people get HIV from kissing?

There has never been a documented case of HIV transmission through kissing.

There may be a small, theoretical risk with kissing, however. The risk with kissing is not with the exchange of saliva. Quantities of virus in saliva

Does AIDS Hurt?

INFORMATION FOR ADULTS

are evidently too small to cause infection. However, if both people have open sores or lesions in the mouth, bleeding gums, or other injuries, it is possible HIV could be transmitted through an exchange of blood. In very vigorous, deep kissing, blood might be drawn, and this also poses a theoretical risk.

Which body fluids carry HIV?

HIV has been found in a number of different body fluids. There are only a few that most of us are likely to come into contact with. These include:
- Blood
- Any body fluid containing visible blood
- Semen
- Vaginal fluids (vaginal or cervical secretions)
- Menstrual blood
- Human breast milk

There are also internal fluids which surround joints, organs or membranes, which carry HIV. Health care workers should take precautions around such fluids, but other people are unlikely to have contact with them.

HIV has also been detected in a few other body fluids, but the concentration of the virus is so small that they are not a danger. We do not need to worry about tears, saliva, urine, feces, vomit, nasal secretions, sputum or sweat, unless visible blood is present.

Can a person become infected with HIV after just one unsafe experience?

Yes. In most cases of sexual transmission or the sharing of needles, people have experienced multiple exposures to HIV before becoming infected. However, there are some cases where a person has become infected after only one unsafe encounter.

INFORMATION FOR ADULTS

Do condoms prevent HIV?

Yes. Latex condoms, properly used, can provide an effective barrier to HIV.

There are instances where condoms may break or slip off. In most cases, these problems are related to "user error." People who are more experienced in the use of condoms are less likely to have problems with breakage and slippage.

What is a latex barrier or latex dam?

A latex barrier is any flat piece of latex that can be used as a barrier during during oral-vaginal or oral-anal sex.

A latex dam is a square of latex about six inches on a side, manufactured for use in dental procedures. You can also make a flat latex barrier by "cutting down" a non-lubricated latex condom (make a cut along the length of the condom and cut off the tip, so it can be rolled out flat).

The flat latex can be placed over the vulva or anus, providing an HIV-resistant barrier for oral sex. No scientific studies have looked at the efficacy of latex barriers in HIV prevention. However, studies have shown that latex condoms are an effective barrier to HIV, and it seems reasonable to believe a "cut down" condom, properly used, will also be effective.

Do sexual lubricants help prevent transmission of HIV?

Lubricants can be helpful in condom use. Properly applied, they can increase the sensation of both partners and decrease incidents of breakage. The lubricant *must* be water-based and water soluble. Any lubricant containing fats or oils (including Crisco, vegetable oil, Vaseline and some commercial sexual lubricants) will break down a latex condom in a matter of seconds.

Some lubricants include spermicides which kill viruses. A common spermicide of this type is nonoxynol-9. A lubricant with nonoxynol 9 may act as a "back up" in case a condom breaks during vaginal or anal intercourse.

INFORMATION FOR ADULTS

However, some individuals have allergic reactions to nonoxynol-9. A rash in the vagina, anus or on the penis would actually increase one's risk of HIV infection because it's easier for the virus to pass through breaks in the skin. Before using any lubricants with nonoxynol-9 for sexual purposes, test the lubricant by rubbing a little on the inside of your arm over a period of several days. If a rash develops, do not use the lubricant.

What is the correct way to clean needles?

The best way to avoid transmission of HIV through needle use is never to share needles or equipment.

If it is necessary to share, flush the equipment liberally with regular household bleach (such as Clorox or Purex), then rinse with water before sharing.

For syringes, draw bleach into the syringe, then expel into the sink or gutter, two times. Then draw water into the syringe, and expel into the sink or gutter, two times.

Is it safe for me and my family to go to the dentist?

Yes. Dentists today are aware of the importance of infection control in the dental office. The only documented cases of HIV transmission within a dental setting all happened at the office of one dentist. No one is sure why this happened, because the dentist himself has since died. However, it is clear that something very unusual and improper took place in these cases.

Dentists and hygienists should wear clean latex gloves during exams and procedures, a face mask (disposable paper type is okay), and glasses or goggles. Large equipment should be wiped down with a disinfectant between patients, and tools used for exams or procedures should be sterilized before reuse.

These protocols are important for the prevention of all diseases, not just HIV. If you have any doubts about your own dentist's office, be sure to ask what the protocol is. Check with your local dental association if you have further questions or need more information.

INFORMATION FOR ADULTS

More Information About HIV and AIDS

The Centers for Disease Control may revise the definition of AIDS. What is the new definition? What impact will this have on the epidemic?

The Centers for Disease Control (CDC) is a federal agency which monitors and studies health practices and disease in the United States. It keeps track of AIDS cases, and developed the definition of AIDS used worldwide today. This definition has been revised twice in the past.

A person is diagnosed with AIDS only if he or she meets certain medical criteria. Until recently, the individual had to have HIV infection and one of several specific conditions or infections associated with HIV. A person with HIV might actually have had many symptoms of illness without qualifying for an AIDS diagnosis, but a person without physical symptoms would not have received an AIDS diagnosis.

In 1992, the definition will probably be changed to take into account certain laboratory values gathered from a type of blood test. The blood test measures the overall health of the immune system, and can indicate whether the immune system is seriously impaired or still functioning well.

This new definition will provide an AIDS diagnosis for many individuals with serious immune system damage who have no physical symptoms, or no severe symptoms, of illness. They may qualify for medical benefits, treatments or social services that were not available to them without an AIDS diagnosis. They may be able to begin early treatments to prevent HIV-associated illnesses or slow the progression of the disease.

What happens to the immune system when someone has HIV?

When a foreign organism enters the body of a person with a healthy immune system, the immune system identifies the intruder, mobilizes defenses against it, and establishes an ongoing specific "watch" to protect against that intruder in the future.

When a person has HIV infection, any part of this sequence may be

INFORMATION FOR ADULTS

disrupted. The immune system may not be able to recognize that a foreign organism has entered the body. If it does, it may be unable to mobilize defenses against it. If the defenses are mobilized, they may not function properly. And finally, the body may be unable to establish a watch system against the intruder in the future.

For example, *Pneumocystis carinii* pneumonia is a common and serious infection in persons with HIV. It is caused by an organism which is all around us. Most of us have been exposed to this organism several times in our lives. With a healthy immune system, the body identifies and overwhelms the organism, and the person never becomes ill with the infection. For a person with HIV, the body may identify the organism, but seems unable to mount an effective defense. The infection takes hold and the person becomes seriously ill.

What is the difference between HIV infection, ARC and AIDS?

Anyone infected with HIV has HIV infection. This might include people with no physical symptoms, people with mild physical symptoms or people with severe physical symptoms.

"ARC" stands for "AIDS-related complex." ARC is an older term that is rarely used today. It described people with symptomatic HIV infection who did not qualify for an AIDS diagnosis.

AIDS is diagnosed in individuals with HIV infection who have developed signs or symptoms of severe immune system impairment. In most cases, people with AIDS are at an advanced stage of HIV infection.

How long can a person be infected with HIV before being diagnosed with AIDS?

The length of time from first infection to diagnosis with AIDS, sometimes called the "incubation period" for AIDS, varies from person to person. In rare cases, it may be as little as a few weeks or months. Some people have had HIV infection for 12 years or longer, and still do not have an AIDS diagnosis. The average length of the incubation period has been

INFORMATION FOR ADULTS

about ten years. The new diagnosis for AIDS may shorten this period slightly.

Is HIV a "death sentence"? Will everyone with HIV die?

For most people with HIV, the condition has been progressive and deteriorative—over time people get sicker, and the immune system becomes increasingly impaired. There are no medically documented cases of people who have recovered from HIV.

However, there are many people living with HIV today who have done well for years, and plan to continue to do well for many more. Out of respect for them, we find it more useful to think of HIV as a "life-threatening" condition rather than as a fatal illness. We hope that one day medical treatments will improve to the point that the progression of disease can be stopped, and we look forward to the day that people with HIV will prevail over their disease and survive the infection.

When will there be a vaccine for HIV?

Vaccine research on HIV has been active for many years, and several vaccines are currently being tested in human trials. An HIV vaccine represents a particular challenge to scientists. So far, there has never been a successful vaccine for a human retrovirus. Any HIV vaccines that seem promising in initial studies will need to go through a long period of testing before becoming generally available. It is likely that it will be many years, at a minimum, before a vaccine is able to be offered.

At the present time, prevention is the only "vaccine" we have, and the only one we can count on for the future.

What treatments are available for HIV? When will there be a cure?

The treatment picture for HIV is better today than it was in the 1980s. A number of medications have been developed which slow progression of HIV. There are also treatments that can help prevent some of the common

INFORMATION FOR ADULTS

illnesses that develop in people with HIV. And there are better treatments for many HIV-associated illnesses once they do develop.

Some people with HIV also use non-Western and nonmedical approaches to address their infection. Acupuncture, herbal and Chinese medicine, homeopathy, visualization, vitamins, and support groups have all been used, sometimes along with traditional Western medicine.

None of these developments represents a "cure," however. A true cure for HIV is certainly many years away, if it is even possible. Our hope is that the treatments will continue to improve, providing better protection for people with HIV and causing fewer side effects, until HIV becomes a manageable condition, much like diabetes or high blood pressure is today.

What is the HIV antibody test?

The HIV antibody test is a simple blood test that can indicate whether an individual has produced antibodies to HIV. It is cheaper, easier and more accurate than a test for actual virus.

If the antibody test result is *positive*, it means that antibodies to HIV were detected, and the individual does have HIV infection. He or she would be capable of transmitting the virus to others in unsafe sexual activities or needle sharing.

If the antibody test result is *negative*, it means that no antibodies to HIV were detected. Either the person is not infected with HIV, or the person is infected but has not yet developed antibodies.

Any time a person is infected with a virus, there is a time lag between the point of infection and the development of antibodies to the virus. This is called the "window period." The window period for development of HIV antibody is usually between two weeks and six months. Rarely, it might be longer.

If an individual has tested negative on the antibody test, but has had some HIV-related risk within the past six months, it would be best to be tested again after the six-month period has passed to be quite confident of the results.

INFORMATION FOR ADULTS

I thought antibodies protected you from disease. If people have antibodies to HIV, why do they get sick?

Antibodies are specialized proteins produced by the immune system to fight diseases. Some antibodies are fully effective. Most people, for example, have mumps only one time in their lives. Their body produced antibodies which prevented any future infection of that type. Antibodies to HIV are only partially effective. They seem able to fight progression of the disease at the outset, but appear to lose their effectiveness after a period of time.

Is the HIV antibody test performed on children?

The HIV antibody test can be performed on children. For newborns of infected mothers, however, the test results are complicated by the presence of maternal serum and maternal antibody in the infant's blood. This means that an infant who tests positive may *not* actually be infected with the virus, but might have antibodies from the mother's blood in its system. This situation usually resolves by the time the child is about 18 months old. The mother's antibodies have cleared from the child's system. Antibody tests after that will be about as reliable as tests on adults.

There are some experimental tests which have helped detect HIV infection in newborns and infants during the first 18 months of life.

How many children have been diagnosed with AIDS? How have they become infected?

At the end of 1991, about 3,500 children (under age 13) had been diagnosed with AIDS. The great majority of these were children of mothers with HIV (about 84 percent). Smaller numbers of children were infected through the use of medicines treating hemophilia (5 percent), through the receipt of a blood transfusion (8 percent), or had an undetermined risk (2 percent).

Children with AIDS may have carried HIV infection for many years before receiving an AIDS diagnosis. This is why we continue to see some new cases of AIDS associated with use of hemophilia medicines or blood

Does AIDS Hurt?

INFORMATION FOR ADULTS

transfusions. However, new cases of HIV infection are now almost solely related to the presence of HIV infection in the mother. Transfusion associated HIV is very rare today, and medicines used to treat hemophilia no longer carry a risk of HIV infection.

Does HIV affect children the same way it affects adults?

Adults with HIV usually look and feel healthy for many years after first becoming infected. Over time, they begin to develop a number of unusual diseases that are not seen in people with healthy immune systems; or they develop unusually severe cases of more common diseases.

Children born with HIV infection tend to develop severe illness early on, often within the first few months of life. They may develop some of the unusual infections seen in adults with immune system problems. They may also develop unusually severe cases of common childhood illnesses.

Earlier, medical providers believed that illness in children with HIV would progress rapidly, and that few of these children would live beyond the early childhood years. Now, we have seen some children who have had HIV infection for a number of years and are still doing very well. While most children with HIV are still expected to have greatly shortened lifespans complicated by severe illness, a few have lived to age ten and beyond without serious health problems.

How serious is the threat of HIV infection of children as a result of sexual molestation?

This is a question we cannot answer with certainty. Our sense is that the likelihood of this occurring is real, but we hope it is relatively small.

Many children are sexually molested. In one study, 28 percent of women surveyed reported being sexually abused before the age of 14. Another recent report suggested that one quarter of all abuse occurs before the age of seven. Boys are molested too. Some current estimates suggest that one in three girls and about one in ten boys are sexually molested before adulthood.

INFORMATION FOR ADULTS

Sexual abuse can be perpetrated by HIV-infected adults. A few such cases are known to have occurred. We are not referring only to the possibility of homosexual men with HIV molesting children. While this is one part of the risk, the molestation of children by heterosexually identified men is far more common and concerns us greatly. We hope parents and communities will be alert to *all* cases of child molestation and the many potential risks involved, and act swiftly to intervene in cases of known or suspected sexual molestation.

How many children with HIV will actually be attending elementary school classes?

This is another question that is difficult to answer. While we can count cases of AIDS among elementary-age children (AIDS cases must be reported to the CDC), we do not have a way of counting children with HIV.

It has been estimated that there may be as many as 20,000 to 30,000 children with HIV in the United States today. If these numbers are accurate, most of these children will be perinatal cases infected at the time of birth. Many children born with HIV will not survive to school age.

However, with earlier identification of HIV infection and better treatments, some children are living longer. Others evidently are not developing serious illnesses in the first place. We suggest that schools prepare themselves for the possibility that children with HIV may be attending classes now or in the future.

Most young children with HIV will be offspring of injection-drug-using parents. I do not think we have those kinds of children in our community.

Drug use and abuse, including injection drug use, cuts across all races, classes and ethnicities. It is present in all communities. Injection drug users may live on the streets, surviving from fix to fix, supporting their habit through criminal activity. But most injection drug users are working people who live in homes and have families.

Even people who only use injection drugs on occasion usually share

INFORMATION FOR ADULTS

needles with others at some point. They are likely to see their use as "recreational" and do not consider it a problem. Since injection drug use is an illegal activity, users are not easy to identify. Denial—of drug dependence and HIV risks—is common and powerful among this population.

We hope as many communities as possible will be spared the tragedy of children being infected with HIV. The risk remains, however, even in communities that are not aware of a significant presence of injection drug users.

What is the likelihood of a young child with HIV passing it on to other students or teachers in school, or to other children or adults participating in a community program?

Remember that HIV transmission can only take place when one individual takes into his or her body the blood, semen or vaginal fluids of another person infected with HIV. Young children are not likely to have this kind of exposure to others in school or community settings.

There is some reasonable concern about the presence of blood in a schoolyard injury. Children should be taught not to touch someone else's blood in the case of an injury, but to call an adult for help.

People often express concerns about a child with HIV fighting with other children, or having open sores. If a child with HIV has significant behavioral problems, or has open sores or lesions which cannot be covered, it may be necessary to keep the child from usual school activities. This would be an exceptional case. Most children with HIV will do well in a school or community setting and do not pose any risk to their peers.

Teachers and others who work with children should be familiar with proper precautions for first aid and cleaning of body fluids. Uniform guidelines for such tasks should be established at all schools and agencies. Latex gloves should be used in response to first-aid situations involving blood. Spills of blood should be cleaned with a 1:10 solution of bleach (1 part bleach to 9 parts water), and vinyl or latex gloves should be worn for

INFORMATION FOR ADULTS

cleaning. Hands should be washed with soap and water after first aid or cleaning.

These guidelines will prevent transmission of HIV and many other diseases.

Doubts About Casual Transmission

I'm not convinced HIV can't be transmitted casually. There is so much we don't know about this disease.

People often have this concern, and it is understandable. HIV is a serious, life-threatening disease. New information is being reported on HIV and AIDS all the time. Government and civic officials often discount worries about casual transmission, but some people do not trust these reassurances.

Remember that we actually know a great deal about HIV. We know it is the cause of AIDS. We know quite a bit about the structure of the virus. We understand how the virus attacks the immune system, and we have seen that it is fragile and dies easily outside the human body. We are familiar now with the progression of disease and the range of illnesses that affects people with HIV.

From studies of thousands of people, we understand that HIV is transmitted only in certain circumstances—most often where blood, semen or vaginal fluids of an infected person enter the body of someone else. There are also some medical situations where the blood, organs or internal body fluids of an infected person have entered the body of someone else and infection has developed.

The information about HIV transmission and prevention has not changed significantly in many years. Most of the new information reported today either refines what we already know about HIV, or addresses issues for which we do not have answers: how to stop the progression of disease in someone infected, how to cure it, how to vaccinate against it, and how to get people to follow prevention guidelines.

INFORMATION FOR ADULTS

People's questions about casual transmission are likely to continue. But a close look at the most common questions reinforces the scientific findings that HIV is not casually transmitted. We review these below.

The incubation period for AIDS might go on for ten years or more. How can you be sure that people who have had casual contact with someone with AIDS are not in that ten-year period of incubation? The disease could appear years from now.

The incubation period for AIDS is the span of time between first infection with HIV and the development of signs or symptoms which qualify for an AIDS diagnosis. It may be ten years or longer in some individuals. This is a long time.

However, the length of time between first infection and the development of HIV antibodies is fairly short, usually occurring in two to twelve weeks, occasionally taking as long as six months. We can test easily for the presence of HIV antibody. If someone had been infected through casual contact, evidence would be available within a short period of time.

Many antibody studies have been performed on family members of people with HIV who share casual contact, and there has never been a spread of infection except where there is a known risk activity—for example, if a man and woman have unprotected sexual intercourse. There have also been studies of residential school settings where some students were known to have HIV. In dozens of such studies carried out worldwide, there has never been evidence of transmission through casual contact.

About 3 percent of AIDS cases in the United States have "no identified risk" for AIDS. Where did these several thousand people get AIDS? Couldn't they have gotten it through casual contact?

Reporting on a disease diagnosed in over 200,000 Americans is a true challenge. Those affected are dispersed over the entire country and are

INFORMATION FOR ADULTS

treated in a variety of medical settings. Of these hundreds of thousands of individuals, 97 percent have a known risk factor.

The Centers for Disease Control (CDC) regularly reviews cases with undetermined risks, looking for further information which can help clarify how a person became infected with HIV. On careful follow-up, most individuals are found to have well-established risk factors (such as sexual contact or needle sharing with an infected individual), or suspected risk factors (such as a history of sexual contact or needle sharing with someone themselves at risk). The reasons the CDC cannot establish risks for other individuals include:

1. The most common risk factors for HIV—sharing injection drug equipment or having unsafe, male-to-male sexual contact—are highly stigmatized activities. Many people are unable or unwilling to admit to these behaviors.
2. Some people visit a medical facility when they are ill and do not return for later follow-up. Diagnostic tests run at the initial visit may result in a diagnosis of AIDS at a later time. Because the individual does not return, no further information can be gathered on the person's risk history.
3. Some people are too ill at the time of an AIDS diagnosis to provide information about themselves.
4. Some individuals are diagnosed with AIDS after death. Risk information is often unavailable in these circumstances.
5. In the past, in a very few instances, individuals who did not actually have AIDS were inappropriately classified as AIDS cases. Refinements in the definition of AIDS have made this an unlikely problem today.

INFORMATION FOR ADULTS

Further Information

I have other questions you have not answered here. Where can I get answers?

You can get your questions about HIV answered through the toll-free National AIDS Hotline.

> English: (800) 342-AIDS (or 342-2437)
> Spanish: (800) 344-SIDA (or 344-7432)
> Deaf Access: (800) 243-7889 (TTD/TTY)

You may also have local resources which can provide you with further information. The National AIDS Hotline can tell you about information resources in your area.

Chapter 11

Staying Updated on HIV Information

News about HIV is always being reported, and often there is a sense that we cannot possibly keep up with all the current knowledge. Many teachers and parents (as well as HIV educators) wonder how well they can teach children about HIV when things change so quickly. It is impressive to consider that in 1981, when the disease was first recognized and described, we did not even know what the cause was. Today, we know AIDS is caused by HIV. We understand how HIV is transmitted; we know how to prevent transmission; we have a good screening test that can protect the blood supply and help people determine whether they are infected; and we have treatments that can help, but not cure, people with HIV.

Scientists will continue to discover new information about HIV, but it is important to remember that the most essential knowledge to share with young children has not changed in many years. HIV is still a serious disease that primarily affects adults. Children rarely engage in the kinds of activities that might transmit HIV. Adults can protect themselves from infection with correct information about HIV. And doctors and scientists the world over are working hard to come up with ways to help people who have HIV.

If we consider the more sophisticated questions some children may have about AIDS transmission and prevention, we see that this information has also remained the same. The modes of transmission described in 1983—sexual intercourse, blood exchange through needle use or other means, and perinatal transmission from mother to fetus—are the only known means of transmission many years and hundreds of thousands of cases later. Prevention strategies—sexual abstinence, mutual monogamy or the practice of safer sex techniques with sexual partners; and abstinence from injection-drug use or not sharing needles—are not any different today than they were nearly ten years ago. The risks for young children overall continue to be very small (except for newborns of injection-drug–using parents), and our main task when young children express concerns about AIDS is to reassure them that they are not at risk of exposure in their usual day to day behaviors.

For this most basic education for young children, neither parents nor teachers need to make any unusual or heroic effort to keep up to date on the most recent scientific advances in HIV research. Major changes in information about HIV as well as updates on the numbers of cases recorded are usually reported in newspapers and news magazines. Regular reading of these sources should keep parents and teachers adequately informed. You can check the sources listed in Section 3, *Further Resources,* for current information or to answer any questions that arise. As children grow and mature, somewhat more effort may be needed in this regard. We would recommend that teachers of older elementary, middle and high school students be updated regularly on HIV information through inservice training, newsletters, school bulletins, professional journals, and so forth.

Chapter 12

HIV Information and Developmental Stages: What Do Children Want to Know About AIDS, When?

As children grow and mature and they face new experiences, different kinds of questions and concerns about HIV will naturally arise. A child who has just turned two is unlikely to have worries about AIDS under any circumstances. A five year old may be quite disinterested in the matter until overhearing a television program or adult conversation in which AIDS is mentioned, then suddenly express great curiosity or concern. A sophisticated ten year old may have a thorough understanding of HIV transmission and prevention.

In this chapter, we review typical issues related to HIV education by age group, and make general suggestions about how to respond to children's questions and needs. *Remember that developmental guidelines are always generalizations, and individual children will vary.* Many different elements affect children's development, among them region (in what part of the country does the child live?), race and ethnicity, language history (is the child being raised in a bilingual family? does the child speak a language at home different from the language used at school?), socioeconomic status, culture, and individual personality.

To set the necessary foundation to educate children well about AIDS, we suggest several general goals:

1. to promote self-esteem and positive self-image, confidence and self-determination for the child

2. to teach the value of health and the idea that personal effort is required to protect one's own health
3. to inform about the basics of human sexuality, drug use and HIV to the extent that this is relevant and appropriate
4. to help children understand the nature of human intimacy and the range of human relationships, again at levels appropriate for the child
5. to provide children with skills necessary to protect them from HIV-related risks
6. to help children develop a sense of belonging and commitment to their communities, and to feel compassion for people affected by the HIV epidemic

Infants (birth to 11 months)

The infant is extremely egocentric and self-involved, relating to other people and the environment primarily in terms of his or her own bodily comfort. Body sensations are the major way the infant experiences the world, and this earliest period is a very sensual one. Constant and loving physical touch is essential to the child's healthy development. Bonds to the family are established, and the major emotional task of the infant is to learn to trust that caretakers will provide a safe and comfortable environment. Infants smile, laugh, cry, establish and hold eye contact, and generally enjoy social attention and people. Boys experience penile erections and girls experience clitoral erections and vaginal lubrication. Most infants, as they develop the necessary muscle coordination, engage in some genital touching and stimulation during bath or other times diapers are removed.

At this stage, children obviously are not asking questions about AIDS or anything else. But in these earliest months of a child's life, the parents are offering important lessons about self-concept and body sensation. If parents restrict children from genital touching, the child understands that genitals are disapproved of. If a child has a chaotic or difficult environment with irregular and unreliable care, he or she cannot learn to trust in caretakers. Without this essential early trust experience, later development of self-trust and self-confidence is difficult. The older child (and teen) with low self-esteem and poor self-concept will not be able to care effectively for personal health and well-being.

A loving, nurturing and accepting environment for an infant lays a foundation for later success in understanding and coping with these issues.

Toddlers

Young toddlers (one year olds) continue to be quite egocentric, but begin for the first time to have a sense of themselves as separate from others. Speech begins and communication skills improve. This child delights in the magical effects of language—if the child says "hi" to someone, that person often responds! Early toddlers usually express many emotions—jealousy, anger, love and attachment. They are intensely interested in the surrounding environment, are active and curious, and explore anything they can get into. Attention shifts rapidly. Play activities are solitary, though the child enjoys watching others at play, work or other pastimes.

Older toddlers (two year olds) are able to focus a bit more, though the attention span is still short. There is a greater sense of individuality and separateness. Self-concept and self-esteem begin to develop, based on the appraisal of the parents and other significant adults in the child's life.

The two year old experiments with limits and boundaries—running away from caretakers, disobeying, being negative. He or she also likes to affect the physical environment. However, in these explorations, the child comes face to face with family rules and the demands of social conformity. He or she learns that independence and freedom are possible only when certain conventions are followed. While the child does not truly understand right from wrong, he or she does respond to consistently applied limits.

Rituals and routines of behavior are very important. Early health practices regarding grooming, bathing and eating are established. Toilet training is accomplished.

Children this age like to help out with tasks and love to do things for themselves. Family relations interest them, and they may act out family experiences in play with other children. If they have fears, these will tend to be of things like giants, monsters or the dark.

Parents and caretakers of both younger and older toddlers can continue providing the loving and secure environment the child needs while beginning to set routines and family rules. As the child grows and develops, the list of routines and rules will lengthen. By promoting (and sometimes enforcing) hygiene practices—brushing teeth, bathing, combing hair—parents teach children that good health is important and it takes some effort to protect it.

The child is learning about intimacy and family relationships. He or she feels differently toward mother and father than a stranger, for example. Behavior allowed with immediate family may differ from behavior accepted around visitors. While this may seem a long way from the complexities of intimate adult sexual relationships, it is this very basic level of understanding that provides a foundation for children to expand on as they mature.

Children also learn names of body parts during this period. Using correct names for genitals (penis, testicles, vagina, vulva, clitoris, urethra) teaches children that there is no shame associated with having genitals. This is one of the earliest and most positive sexuality education tasks of parents.

Toddlers do not understand concepts of past, present or future, nor do they have the tools necessary to conceptualize the passage of time.

Children this age may pick up slang words describing sexual practices or excretory functions, or they may repeat the word "AIDS" if they have heard it somewhere. If adults act startled or upset at these times, the child may repeat the words because he or she enjoys watching this reaction. A neutral response from adults will send the child in search of different, more exciting words to use. There is no particular meaning for a two year old in such language. AIDS is well beyond this child's comprehension.

Early Childhood

Three years: Three year olds develop more amenable social skills. They enjoy being affectionate with other children and adults, are often friendly and agreeable, learn to share toys and enjoy being with their peers. Like their younger counterparts, they experience powerful emotions, but they are learning skills of self-control and restraint, which help them cope with these feelings more effectively. Sibling rivalry becomes apparent at this age.

By three years, children can understand the anatomical differences between the sexes and are reassured by positive, basic explanations of the normalcy and health of both girls' and boys' genitalia. There may be some display of sexual organs in play with other children and removing of clothes outdoors. These children are curious about the different postures boys and girls use for urinating, and girls will often try to urinate standing up.

Three year olds are also interested in babies and like to see and be around infants. Questions about where babies come from may first arise at this age.

Parental attentions can continue to teach the three year old self-confidence, norms of social behavior and adherence to rules. At this age, as children socialize more with peers, they also share sexual information with one another. Parents who have been careful and factual in their sexuality education and terminology may be surprised by some of the ideas and words their children come home with. Ongoing dialogue and willingness to answer questions becomes important, and will continue to be important throughout the child's development to adulthood. Where caretakers see or hear obvious sexual misinformation, they may wish to bring up the topic and correct misunderstandings. There will continue to be a fair amount of interest in anatomy and conception, and many opportunities for discussion will usually arise.

Three year olds may develop some interest in death if a pet dies or as they come across dead animals or bugs in their outdoor explorations. They cannot understand the full meaning of death, or its permanence. They often expect dead beings to "wake up again" and get on with the things they normally do—"The bird has flown back to the sky now," they might say, ignoring the decomposing corpse on the ground nearby. Health and well-being are abstract concepts that will not make much sense to a three year old, but caretakers can use such concepts in talking about hygiene and health habits, and the child will "grow" into them ("I want you to eat more of your vegetables before you eat your cookie. You need lots of 'grow food' to stay healthy.") Mild illness will not stop this child, though moderate or severe illness is certainly noted. Illness in others is not especially important except if it might affect the child quite directly—"Your mother is sick and trying to sleep. Please be quiet and don't disturb her." Three year olds will not be interested in AIDS.

Four years: Four year olds continue to be fairly cooperative, though they are also selfish and impatient. They play imaginative games with peers and may have a make-believe playmate. They enjoy the companionship of children more than adults, while continuing to develop strong feelings of love and attachment to their family and home. They talk openly with others about family events, including things parents would prefer to keep private!

This child is proud of accomplishments, enjoys praise, and is sensitive to blame. He or she likes to brag and boast, is beginning to understand concepts of "good" and "bad," and has the capacity for some self-criticism. "Privacy" can be explained to the child, and rules about respecting others' privacy can be followed. Four year olds also enjoy having some privacy of their own and can be taught about personal activities that are best carried out privately (for example, toileting or masturbation).

The four year old is clear about and wants to state his or her gender identity: "I am a girl and you are a boy." There is interest in human bodies generally, especially how males and females are different, what the parts of the body usually covered by clothes look like, how adults differ from children and whether children will look like their parents when they grow up. Questions about the origins of babies will continue, including how a baby gets out of its mother's "stomach."

The four year old continues to benefit from parental love and guidance, and the willingness of caretakers to answer questions about people, sexuality and reproduction. A mature four year old with a reasonable foundation of knowledge about the anatomical differences between males and females is capable of understanding a simple explanation of intercourse. Some children will ask these kinds of questions, others will not. Some children this age may ask about AIDS, but most will not. For most four year olds, health will continue to be an abstract and not especially relevant concept, though there is interest in *healing*, especially if a wound requires the attention of a bandage. Concepts about death continue to be vague, with little understanding of either a biologic or spiritual meaning of death.

The four year old is knowledgeable about family rules and generally follows them, but may not have a clear understanding of the basis for the rules. Self-care and self-protection are still practiced primarily out of habit and to accommodate adults. These children understand that they are not to cross the street without holding a grown-up's hand, or go anywhere with strangers.

Adults may carry on conversations while children pursue other pastimes nearby and appear not to be listening. In fact, children often *do* listen carefully to these grown-up discussions. By age four, they will be learning a great deal from "overheard" conversations. Parents especially can take advantage of this by pursuing discussions that will contribute appropriately to a child's knowledge and sense of well-being, whether this be about health generally, human sexuality or other relevant topics. Such conversations can serve as a reinforcement of earlier discussions with a child, or might help set some basis for future talk.

School Age

Five years: Beginning school is an important transition for children and their families. While many children attend daycare and preschool facilities, most will find themselves in the less intimate and more structured setting of public school around age five. A whole new realm of influence and experience enter both the child's and the family's life.

Many five year olds talk constantly and are interested in everything. They are more attentive to their surroundings and hear things they might have ignored when they were younger. They bring home new words, new concepts and challenging questions which may startle or baffle parents. Often these have to do with human sexuality. It is an exciting, rewarding and sometimes difficult time for all.

The five year old is blossoming in social skills. He or she wants to please parents, teachers and other important adults, likes to make friends, and is learning more about leadership, giving and receiving, and social convention. This child is protective of younger children and concerned about the welfare of others. He or she spends more time with playmates than with family, and is increasingly more autonomous. There is tremendous motivation to grow up, be as big as parents, or act like older kids.

Five year olds are fairly independent in most of their health and grooming routines, and they generally understand and follow safety rules well. At this age, children seem to have limitless energy. They enjoy showing off their vigor, strength and health. Mild illness will hardly slow them—they are frustrated by grown-ups' attempts to calm them down when they run a temperature or have a cough.

Many concerns relevant to HIV are of interest to the five year old: conception, birth, marriage, death, sexuality and all kinds of human relationships. Fears are often much more specific than for the younger child. Five year olds fear things like violent death, kidnapers and criminals. Fears of fatal diseases or AIDS specifically may arise for some five year olds. The concept of health as a state of strength and energy is willingly accepted. In his or her attempt to catch up with adults, the five year old may well pronounce, "I am strong and healthy and powerful!" Germs are attributed as the cause of many diseases, though there may be genuine confusion about what germs really are, what they look like and where they hide. This child understands that colds and flu can be passed by kissing or sharing cups. Rules, which were once followed from blind obedience, may now be followed because they are rational and useful.

With a five year old, parents, caretakers and teachers will have many opportunities to teach about family relationships, other human relationships, health practices, community responsibilities and sexuality. Human reproduction, simply explained, is understood by most five year olds (though they may forget correct explanations and continue with fantasy ideas of babies being manufactured or bought in stores). With this knowledge in place, HIV transmission can be comfortably and appropriately explained to a five year old if necessary. ("Remember how we have talked about how some grown-ups have sexual intercourse? Some illnesses can be passed from one person to another person when people have sexual intercourse. AIDS can be passed this way.")

At this age, questions about AIDS are more likely to arise than before. Children may pursue detailed answers by asking more and more specific questions. This is typical of how five year olds learn—from the general to the specific—and they will do this with any topic of interest.

Six years: The six year old continues with many of the same interests as the five year old. As cognitive skills develop, the six year old is able to handle a wider variety of information at more sophisticated levels. The younger child was interested in events and experiences primarily as they related to him or her personally. The six year old begins to be interested in the experiences of others and to have some empathic awareness even if not directly affected by an event.

Questions about sexuality will continue to be asked at home if the child has felt comfortable doing so thus far. Parents are sometimes surprised to find issues they thought were adequately explained in the past coming up again. Young children tend to remember this information selectively, however, and even very bright children may need explanations repeated several times during this period of their lives.

Children are also aware of other resources for sex information and will certainly explore these avenues as well—peers at school, older siblings, or older students carry a wealth of sexual information of wildly variable accuracy. Television programs or popular music may be suggestive without being thorough. There may be significant confusion about sexual issues.

Some six year olds have developed cognitive skills that allow new kinds of abstraction in thinking about human relationships and life and death. It is around this age that some children will first be able to see that death is a final, irreversible process. There may be further interest in the spiritual implications of life and death.

As the child grows and social contacts in school and other settings expand, there will be increasing likelihood that he or she will hear information about AIDS. A common misconception at this time is that people get AIDS from being bad. Many other beliefs may be inaccurate or magical, and they may change with some frequency.

Seven and eight years: The seven or eight year old continues the trend of growing sophistication in understanding the world, and growing autonomy and independence. Increasingly more time is spent with peers and away from family, and there may be tremendous exposure to television programs, movies and videos full of intriguing information about sexuality, violence and death. Around this age, boys and girls will divide into separate groups on the playground.

These children have longer attention spans; a good orientation to past, present, and future; an understanding of ways of measuring time; and a better ability to remember information after one or two explanations. They are more likely to be able to comprehend death as a permanent event, though this may be complicated by the constant resurrections of dead characters in televisions and videos. They can understand more complicated human relationships, and are themselves beginning to engage in some of the greater complexities of human interaction—they may have a best friend, they may compete with others for the friendship of a popular child, there will usually be particular children they clearly dislike, and they may be hurt deeply in conflicts with their peers.

Interest in sexual matters continues. For some children, there will be more emphasis now on sexual feelings than on curiosity about reproduction. Beginning at birth, children have sexual feelings of their own, and by age seven or eight they may make the connection between what they are feeling and what everyone else is talking about. This is also a time when children who have been open with their parents about their sexual questions in the past might become more private, embarrassed or withdrawn.

Interest in matters other than sexuality continues as well. World events, nuclear arms, poverty, drug use, war and violence all enter the awareness of young children. Questions are raised and anxieties may be expressed when major events or personal experiences bring these kinds of concerns closer to the child's own life. Stories about children with AIDS who have been mistreated may be especially interesting and/or disturbing to these children. Given an opportunity to discuss AIDS with a trustworthy adult, children this age may have many questions, usually over a much broader range of concerns than the five or six year old.

Parents and teachers can offer informative answers to children's questions, and in addition may also seek to impart skills to help children cope with this increasingly difficult information and keep it in healthy perspective in their lives.

Nine and ten years: Nine and ten year olds stand on the threshold of adolescence. Differences in cognitive, social and emotional development, so evident throughout the childhood years, become even more pronounced at this time. Some of these children continue to think and act very concretely, to play children's games, and to enjoy a lot of intimacy with their families. Others are really more like early adolescents, paying attention to styles of dress, dance and music, and spending very little time at play. They may distance themselves more from their families, sometimes having conflicts with parents concerning behavior or values.

Reading becomes an important activity for many children this age. They can involve themselves in full novels, thereby bringing a new dimension to their knowledge of the world. They are able to escape the people and places around them without ever leaving their chairs.

Nine and ten year olds have a better cognitive understanding of cause-and-effect relationships, and are usually capable of understanding a fuller range of human activities as well. They are more tolerant of ambiguity and less insistent on black-and-white solutions, though they still feel most comfortable with concrete answers to questions and problems. Complicated statements and relationships make more sense—this child is much better able to understand, for example, that HIV can be transmitted several different ways.

Ten year olds are quite able to understand that there is a variety of human sexual activities, that there are consequences to sexual behavior (unwanted pregnancy, sexually transmitted disease, emotional difficulties), and that it is a good idea to delay intercourse. It will be important for these children to understand the dangers of HIV, how it is transmitted and how to prevent transmission. They will develop a much more sophisticated understanding of drug abuse problems. In some areas, nine and ten year olds will know older children who are already using substances. It is during these years that many children will have their first real-life practice in turning down offers to use drugs or be sexually active.

These are essential years for parents and other adults to be actively involved with children, to talk with them regularly, to be available to discuss problems and concerns, and to help them strengthen their own sense of self-worth and self-esteem. It is particularly important that children at this age be prepared with sound information and strong personal support to face the increasingly adult demands that await them.

 ❧ ❧ ❧

Ideally, families of children six to ten years old will have regular and ongoing discussions about a whole range of sensitive issues, including human sexuality, personal morality and values. Parents are the most influential teachers of values to children, whether or not they pursue this task deliberately. Children learn from their parents what sorts of values to place on friendships, human beings generally, family and community responsibilities, work, the status of women, the importance of love and intimacy and appropriate roles for children and adults.

Young children love to talk about deep issues (usually for brief periods of time) and to be taken seriously. Questions about HIV and other issues may be searching and thoughtful in these years. Concern for the welfare of others and interest in community values grows. When adults carry on these conversations so that the child understands the content and feels respected, the child is able to develop essential qualities of self-worth and self-confidence.

Classroom teachers can offer structured lessons in health, disease, and how to prevent illness; drug abuse prevention; healthy behaviors concerning diet, sleep and exercise; and different types of human relationships. Children can be helped to develop skills in asking questions and getting answers about things of interest to them. Child sexual abuse prevention programs should be available for first graders and older children. Drug prevention programs are also appropriate at this age, and the role of injection-drug use in the spread of disease (including HIV) can be understood. If a particular school or district has a comprehensive family life education program, this will further help teachers and parents in discussing many of the concerns that arise for young children, including concerns about AIDS and HIV.

The most important thing to keep in mind as you think about talking about HIV/AIDS or other sensitive issues with children is that, while it is a challenging task, it is not difficult when a foundation of knowledge and openness is already set. If an eight year old with no familiarity with human sexuality, health practices or communicable disease asks, "How do people get AIDS?", the answer will be complicated, long and probably confusing for the child. You would need to cover what AIDS is, something about how diseases are passed generally, human sexual practices, the possibility of HIV or other diseases being passed sexually, injection-drug use, and the role of injection drugs in HIV transmission. However, if you have already been talking about these general topics with a child even as young as five, the answer is fairly simple (you can read our example in Chapter 3: *What Are Children Asking and How Can You Answer Them?*).

Chapter 13

Signs of Child Sexual Abuse

Discussions about AIDS may raise particular anxieties for children who have been abused sexually. There are a number of physical and behavioral clues that suggest a child may be a victim of sexual abuse. We include a list of these here to remind parents, teachers and others who provide care to children to always be alert to this possibility.

If you have clear evidence that a child is being abused, we urge you to act swiftly to inform the necessary authorities and see that the child is protected. If you suspect such abuse may be occurring but you are not certain, your local child protective agency will be able to provide you with further advisement. Anonymous calls to these agencies are always possible. You will find them listed in the phone book under "City and County Services." You can also get further information from your local police department.

Indicators of Sexual Abuse in Children*

The following physical and behavioral characteristics may be signaling that a child is a victim of sexual abuse. As with other lists of symptoms, some of the

*Reprinted from *The Educator's Guide to Preventing Child Sexual Abuse*, edited by Mary Nelson and Kay Clark. Santa Cruz, CA: ETR Associates, 1986.

same signs may indicate other types of problems. Until recently, sexual abuse was not often considered as a possible reason for erratic or problem behavior. It is important to recognize that sexual abuse is a possibility when a child/adolescent exhibits several of the following behaviors.

Physical Signs

Bruising, bleeding or infections in the genital/anal area. Physical symptoms may be manifested as difficulty in walking, sitting or urinating; scratching or tugging at clothing around the genital area; torn, stained or bloody clothing; genito-urinary complaints or infections.

There may be no physical indicators that a child is being abused.

Behavioral/Attitudinal Signs

- Eating, sleeping and eliminating disturbances
- Recurrent physical complaints, such as abdominal pain
- Withdrawn or aggressive behavior
- Tired, lethargic, sleepy appearance
- Fearful or suspicious of adults
- Sexually explicit language or behavior not appropriate to the child's age
- Regressive behavior such as whining, excessive crying, thumbsucking, wetting or soiling self
- Aversion to a particular person, place or situation
- Change in school performance, truancy
- Fear, worry, overly serious, depressed
- Anger toward or dislike of adults, authority figures
- Running away from home
- Suicide threats or attempts
- Behavioral defiance, sexual promiscuity, prostitution
- Shy, withdrawn, overburdened appearance
- Substance abuse that is more than experimental
- Reluctance to undress for physical education
- Stealing, shoplifting
- Pregnancy wishes
- Interest in early marriage

- Attraction to older men or dislike of men
- Excessive hand washing, bathing
- Unreasonably restricted social activities or overly protective father
- Poor self-image, low self-esteem
- Fantasies about victimization or violence
- Alienation from family members, rejection of typical family affection
- Fear of strange men and/or strange situations
- Fear of being alone
- Overly clinging or dependent behavior
- Extreme avoidance of touch
- Abrupt change in behavior or personality
- Extreme over-achiever

SECTION 3

FURTHER RESOURCES

Appendix A

Readings

General AIDS Information

Hein, K., and T.F. Digeronimo. 1991. *AIDS: Trading Fears for Facts.* Yonkers, NY: Consumer Reports Books.

Institute of Medicine and National Academy of Sciences. 1980. Revised 1988. *Confronting AIDS: Directions for Public Health, Health Care and Research.* Washington, DC: National Academy Press.

Koop, C.E. 1986. *Surgeon General's Report on Acquired Immune Deficiency Syndrome.* Washington, DC: U.S. Department of Health and Human Services.

Monette, P. 1988. *Borrowed Time: An AIDS Memoir.* New York: Avon Books.

Ruskin, C. 1988. *The Quilt: Stories from the Names Project.* New York: Pocket Books.

Shilts, R. 1988. *And the Band Played On: Politics, People and the AIDS Epidemic.* New York: Penguin Books.

Child Development/Parenting

Boston Women's Health Book Collective. 1978. *Ourselves and Our Children: A Book By and For Parents.* New York: Random House.

Caplan, F. 1985. *The First Twelve Months of Life.* New York: Bantam Books.

Caplan, F., and T. Caplan. 1985. *The Second Twelve Months of Life.* New York: Bantam Books.

Caplan, T., and F. Caplan. 1984. *The Early Childhood Years: The 2 to 6 Year Old.* New York: Bantam Books.

Child Sex Education by Parents and in Schools

Calderone, M., and J. Ramey. 1982. *Talking with Your Child About Sex: Questions and Answers for Children from Birth to Puberty.* New York: Ballentine Books.

Planned Parenthood Federation of America. 1986. *How to Talk With Your Child About Sexuality.* Garden City, NY: Doubleday & Company.

SIECUS (Sex Information and Education Council of the United States). 1991. Guidelines for Comprehensive Sexuality Education: Kindergarten-12th Grade. New York: SIECUS.

Tiffany, J., D. Tobias, R. Arzeymah and J. Zeigler. 1991. *Talking with Kids About AIDS: A Program for Parents and Other Adults Who Care.* Ithaca, NY: Cornell University.

Wilson, P. M. 1991. *When Sex Is the Subject.* Santa Cruz, CA: ETR Associates.

Children's Attitudes Toward Chronic Illness and Death

Grollman, E.A. 1990. *Talking About Death: A Dialogue Between Parent and Child.* Boston: Beacon Press.

Krementz, J. 1989. *How It Feels to Fight for Your Life: The Inspiring Stories of Fourteen Children Who Are Living with Chronic Illness.* New York: Simon & Schuster.

Krementz, J. 1988. *How It Feels When a Parent Dies.* New York: Alfred A. Knopf.

Rando, T. 1984. *Grief, Dying and Death: Clinical Interventions for Caregivers.* Champaign, IL: Research Press Company. [Especially Chapter 12—"The Family of the Dying Patient," and Chapter 13—"The Dying Child."]

Siebert, D., J. Drolet and J. Fetro. In press. *Educating Young Children About Death.* Santa Cruz, CA: ETR Associates.

The Center for Attitudinal Healing. 1979. *There Is a Rainbow Behind Every Dark Cloud.* Millbrae, CA: Celestial Arts.

Family Life Education Curricula for Elementary School Settings

Brown, J., et al. 1984. *Sexuality Education: A Curriculum for Parent/Child Programs*. Santa Cruz, CA: ETR Associates.

DeSpelder, L., and A. Strickland. 1982. *Family Life Education: Resources for the Elementary Classroom, Grades 4, 5 and 6*. Santa Cruz, CA: ETR Associates.

Comprehensive Health Education Materials

American Health Foundation. 1980. *Know Your Body*. New York: American Health Foundation.

National Center for Health Education. 1986. *Growing Healthy, K-6*. New York: National Center for Health Education.

Pollock, M. B., and K. Middleton. 1984. *Elementary School Health Instruction*. St. Louis MO: Times Mirror/Mosby. (Second edition forthcoming.)

Preventing Child Sexual Abuse

Fay, J. 1979. *He Told Me Not to Tell: A Parent's Guide for Talking to Your Child About Sexual Assault*. Renton, WA: King County Rape Relief.

Plummer, C. A. 1984. *Preventing Sexual Abuse: Activities and Strategies for Those Working With Children and Adolescents*. Holmes Beach, FL: Learning Publications, Inc.

Preventing Drug Abuse

Comprehensive Health Education Foundation. 1986. *Here's Looking At You 2000*. Seattle, WA: Comprehensive Health Education.

U.S. Department of Education. 1990. Growing Up Free: A Parent's Guide to Prevention. Washington, DC: U.S. Department of Education.

AIDS and Schools

Centers for Disease Control. 1988. Guidelines for Effective School Health Education to Prevent the Spread of AIDS. *Morbidity and Mortality Weekly Report* 37 (suppl. no. S-2). Atlanta, GA: Centers for Disease Control.

Hooper, S., and G. Gregory. 1986. *AIDS and the Public Schools*. Alexandria, VA: National School Boards Association.

Kirp, D.L. 1989. *Learning by Heart: AIDS and School Children in America's Communities.* New Brunswick, NJ: Rutgers University Press.

Quackenbush, M., M. Nelson and K. Clark, eds. 1988. *The AIDS Challenge: Prevention Education for Young People.* Santa Cruz, CA: ETR Associates.

Talking with Children About Difficult Topics

Dumas, L.S. 1992. *Talking with Your Child About a Troubled World.* New York: Fawcett Columbine.

Centers for Disease Control. 1989. *America Responds to AIDS: AIDS Prevention Guide for Parents and Other Adults Concerned About Youth.* Atlanta, GA: Centers for Disease Control.

Appendix B

Information Sources

The network of AIDS information and service resources is large. There are organizations or agencies responsible for coordinating AIDS services in every state. The national information number, listed below, maintains up-to-date listings of local resources throughout the country. Not all of these organizations have information hotlines.

Hotlines
National AIDS Hotline (toll free)
(800) 342-AIDS—Information in English
(800) 344-SIDA—Information in Spanish
Administered by the American Social Health Association

National Gay Task Force
AIDS Information Hotline
(800) 221-7044
(212) 807-6016 (NY State)

STD National Hotline
(800) 227-8922
Administered by the American Social Health Association

Written Resources: Pamphlets, Brochures, Posters

Call or write for description of materials and price list. Some of these agencies will also provide speakers for school assemblies, consultation for teachers or education for parents.

American Red Cross
AIDS Education Office
1730 D St., NW
Washington, DC 20006
(202) 737-8300
or contact local Red Cross

ETR Associates
P.O. Box 1830
Santa Cruz, CA 95061-1830
(800) 321-4407

Gay Men's Health Crisis, Inc.
132 West 24th St.
New York, NY 10011
(212) 807-6655

Impact AIDS
3692 18th Street
San Francisco CA 94110
(415) 861-3397
Fax (415) 621-3951

National AIDS Information Clearinghouse
P.O. Box 6003
Rockville MD 20850
(800) 458-5231

National AIDS Network
1012 14th St. NW, Suite 601
Washington, DC 20005
(202) 347-0390

U.S. Public Health Service
Public Affairs Office
Hubert H. Humphrey Building , Room 725-H
200 Independence Ave., SW
Washington, DC 20201
(202) 245-6867

About the Authors

Marcia Quackenbush, MS, MFCC, is Coordinator of Special Projects for the AIDS Health Project, a program of the University of California, San Francisco, and the San Francisco Department of Public Health. She has been active in AIDS prevention education for youth since early 1984. She has trained teachers and other educators on AIDS prevention approaches with children and youth, and is coauthor of *Teaching AIDS*, a resource guide for secondary teachers. In her role as an advocate for AIDS education, she has appeared on national television, spoken on radio shows across the country, and testified before a Congressional Committee. She counsels persons with AIDS and HIV infection and has a private practice in psychotherapy.

Sylvia F. Villarreal, MD, is Assistant Clinical Professor of Pediatrics and a staff member of the Children's Health Center at San Francisco General Hospital. She is Director of the Kempe High Risk Clinic and Early Childhood Services. Her community work includes membership on the San Francisco Mayor's HIV Health Services Planning Council. She is a member of the board of directors for the California Children's Lobby. Dr. Villarreal has published extensively on health care issues and her field of research is nonorganic failure to thrive.

Tackle Today's Tough Issues With More Practical Handbooks

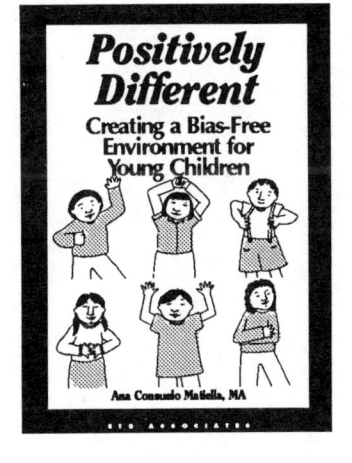

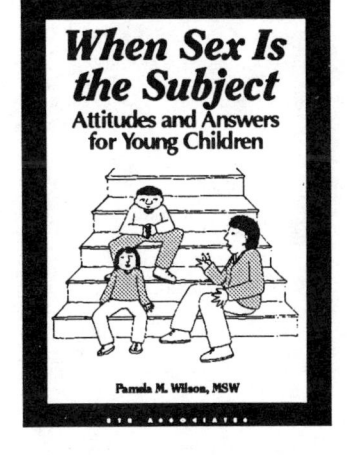

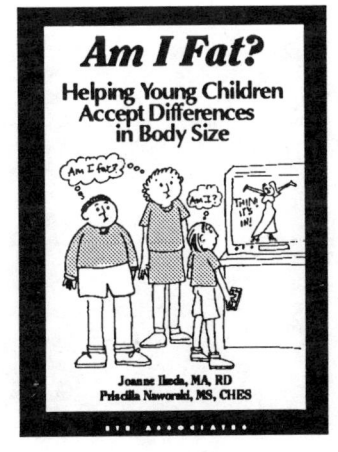

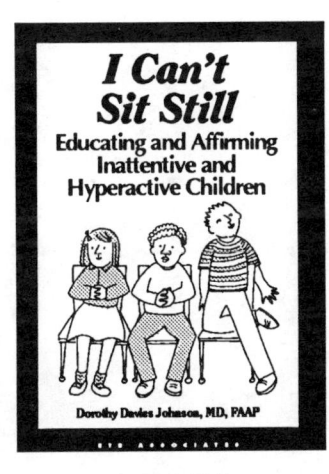

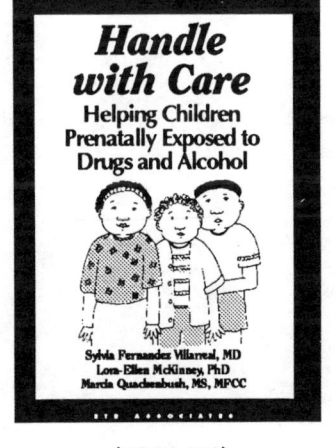

Positively Different
Creating a Bias-Free Environment for Young Children
Ana Consuelo Matiella, MA
(#509-H1)

When Sex Is the Subject
Attitudes and Answers for Young Children
Pamela M. Wilson, MSW
(#583-H1)

Am I Fat?
Helping Young Children Accept Differences in Body Size
Joanne Ikeda, MA, RD
Priscilla Naworski, MS, CHES
(#569-H1)

I Can't Sit Still
Educating and Affirming Inattentive and Hyperactive Children
Dorothy Davies Johnson, MD, FAAP
(#560-H1)

Handle with Care
Helping Children Prenatally Exposed to Drugs and Alcohol
Sylvia Fernandez Villarreal, MD
Lora-Ellen McKinney, PhD
Marcia Quackenbush, MS, MFCC
(#594-H1)

Learn a variety of positive, hands-on approaches to help children up to age ten understand the health issues that shape their lives. The Issues Books from ETR Associates. For more information and a complete list of Issues Books...

Call Toll-Free 1 (800) 321-4407

or contact:
**Sales Department
ETR Associates**
P.O. Box 1830
Santa Cruz, CA 95061-1830
FAX: (408) 438-4284